THE
YOGA
THING

THE
YOGA
THING

The Easy, Practical Way
to Enjoy
Physical Well-Being
and Freedom from Stress,
Anxiety, and Fatigue

by Nancy Roberts

Photographs by Keith Roberts

HAWTHORN BOOKS, INC.
W. CLEMENT STONE, PUBLISHER
New York

To Mama,
with love and appreciation
for a lifetime
of positive programming

Contents

Foreword

It is my great pleasure to write a short foreword to a book on yoga written by my own pupil, Nancy Roberts, particularly since her book is extremely well written.

A yoga teacher has, in a way, a greater responsibility than a teacher in any other field since he or she has to deal not only with the physical, but also with the moral, mental, and spiritual aspects of the students. It is, therefore, extremely important to have a good yoga instructor. And Nancy Roberts is such an instructor. She has completed our Spiritual Advancement of the Individual (S.A.I.) Foundation's Annual Teachers' Course and holds the Teacher's Certificate, which is issued after one passes the examinations.

During my many years of teaching yoga and training yoga instructors, I have seen yoga's rapid rise in popularity and recognition throughout this country and the rest of the world. One of my greatest concerns is that the name of this ancient Indian science and art of living not be spoiled, nor its high ideals and standards lowered. True yoga can be accurately presented only by properly trained and qualified instructors, and not by the half-baked, self-styled ones who distort the real meaning of this oldest system of personal development.

The Yoga Thing is written with precision and knowledge of the subject, and should be well received by those interested in yoga. In it the reader will find clear explanations and photographs of the asanas (yoga postures), and much useful and practical advice. It contains as well a great deal of information about other methods not directly related to yoga, but also dealing with the expansion of the human mind.

Best wishes for the success of this book from the heart of

INDRA DEVI
Founder President
Spiritual Advancement
of the Individual (S.A.I.)
Foundation, Inc.

"Sai Nilayam"
Tecate, California

1

AN OVERVIEW:
WHAT IS THE YOGA THING?

Yoga is an ancient art and science designed for the realization of human potential. This giant body of information and wisdom stands with its feet rooted in the India that existed before Christ and yet has its eyes fixed firmly on the stars of tomorrow. It has withstood the test of time and now is leading twentieth-century scientists in their search for a better understanding of the nature of man.

As a system of physical fitness it is incomparably practical, but its greatest value is for those who know that there is much more to life than what can be measured, tested, analyzed, and proved—for those who know that looking at a man is like looking at an iceberg: What you see is only a minute portion of what is there.

If you've never given yoga a second thought, now might be the time to do so, for it appeals to even those who normally hate the idea of exercise. If you're tense, it will teach you to relax; if you can't touch your toes, it will make you more flexible—physically and mentally—and if you have a low threshold of boredom, it has 84,000 posture variations to hold your attention. And although yoga science can provide guidelines for all areas of life, you can take as much or as little as you choose. If you merely wish to shape up, slim down, and feel better, yoga can show you how. But if your interests are deeper, if you're seeking the spiritual path, it's all there.

This ancient Oriental discipline, not quite a religion and not just a physical-fitness regime, is sweeping the country at a time when our technological advances are producing unprecedented breakthroughs in all areas of knowledge and information. Our fast-paced twentieth century is also producing a society in which alcoholism and drug addiction are primary health problems, tension is almost epidemic, and the ability to relax is a lost art.

It may be that such intensely personal, introspective movements as yoga, encounter groups, and now alphagenics (getting to know your own brain waves) are an instinctive effort at self-preservation, or preservation of that inner core of individuality that is the self. Perhaps it's another example of Newton's third law of motion—that for every action there is an equal and opposite reaction: the more we probe outer space, the more we probe, correspondingly, inner space—a microcosmic balancing act that people turn to when their outer environment expands too rapidly for comfort.

The word "yoga" used to conjure up images of fakirs lying on a bed of nails or walking barefoot over burning coals and was pretty much in the same bag as the snake charmers, mystics, and the oddballs of the spook world. It is, in fact, none of these. In its simplest form yoga is a system of physical, mental, and spiritual development.

Because our knowledge explosion is so vast, and our lives so fast-paced, the yoga method that develops latent potential and instills a feeling of personal worth and individuality is particularly welcome. Any system that does this, along with streamlining the body, calming the nerves, and retarding the aging process, is bound to attract a following.

The concept of physical fitness is not a new one. During the Kennedy administration physical fitness became the watchword, and the establishment of the President's Council on Physical Fitness assured instant success for exercise booklets such as the R.C.A.F. Basic Exercise Program and other similar shape-up literature. We've also had isometrics and isotonics and the jogging craze, followed by sauna shorts. Many people turned on to these concepts have since tuned out because they found the routines so boring. Nearly everyone has participated in an exercise program of sorts at some time, but relatively few have made calisthenics a permanent part of their lives.

Yoga devotees, on the other hand, turn to this form of exercise for physical reasons but remain turned on because it is the only program that involves the entire individual—physically, mentally, and spiritually. That this yoga movement comes at a time when organized religion, as such, is faltering could indicate that people are groping their way back to self-reliance instead of dependence on outside factors for support or salvation.

Self-reliance is one of the basic attributes on which this country was founded. Today's swingers are probably unaware that the admonition

"Do your own thing" is a direct steal from Ralph Waldo Emerson's essay "Self-Reliance" written back in the dark ages—in 1841. Surprisingly, Emerson and his transcendentalist cronies—Henry David Thoreau, Bronson Alcott, and Walt Whitman—were America's first gurus.*

There are several branches of yoga, and all have the same ultimate purpose: the uniting of man, the finite, with the infinite, whether this be called God, truth, light, cosmic consciousness, or ultimate reality. Translated into simpler terms, the purpose of all yoga is self-realization. While Emerson and his Concord group actually espoused raja-yoga, the "kingly" yoga, today's gurus are disseminating hatha-yoga, that which is concerned with physical and mental well-being.

The goals of hatha-yoga are realized through a combination of exercises, called asanas, or postures, controlled breathing, diet, and relaxation. The postures are designed to stretch and activate every muscle in the body. Gymnastics and calisthenics do this and only this, which is much like taking care of the outside of an automobile and forgetting about the engine. Yoga goes further in that its postures affect all the bodily functions—circulation, elimination, digestion, and the endocrine and nervous systems.

Another basic premise of yoga is that there is a definite link between mind and body—that whatever affects the body affects the mind and whatever affects the mind affects the body. This awareness of the mind's power has been another primary difference between yoga and calisthenics. You can do push-ups and worry about your job at the same time, but when you do a yoga posture, your mind is focused on what the posture is doing for you internally and externally.

The Power of the Mind

The power of the mind has been largely ignored by Western cultures which are so geared to tangibility, to that which can be tested, analyzed, measured, and proved. Despite the fact that such books as Norman Vincent Peale's *The Power of Positive Thinking* have been national best-sellers, the importance of mind power has not caught on with the masses. The medical profession, however, is becoming increasingly aware of the tremendous role the mind plays in human health.

The word "yoga" comes from the Sanskrit word *yuj*, which means union or to join, and initially referred to the joining of the physical, mental, and spiritual components in man. On a higher plane it signified the union of

* The first syllable, *gu*, in Sanskrit, means darkness; the second syllable, *ru*, means light. A guru is a spiritual teacher who leads the student from darkness to light.

man and God. Twentieth-century yoga is assuming an added dimension and may be the unifying factor between the mystical East and the materialistic West. The United States Government and the medical profession are cast in the unlikely role of marriage brokers in this East-West union. Hopefully, the offspring of this marriage may be an era in which man himself controls his own heart rate, blood pressure, body temperature, and other functions long thought to be involuntary.

The yogis of India, who have for centuries claimed to control all bodily functions at will, are now being studied by such research organizations as the Menninger Foundation in Topeka, Kansas, via grants from the U.S. Department of Health, Education, and Welfare. The object of this research is biofeedback training, which may revolutionize the medical profession by curing illness through mind control instead of medicine.

A primary subject in this research is Swami Rama, a fascinating fortyish yogi from India who has been tested extensively at the Menninger Foundation. During these tests, which were electronically monitored, the swami stopped his heart for seventeen seconds, raised the temperature in one hand by 15° and then reversed it, and moved a metal bar thirty degrees simply by concentrating on it. The metal bar, incidentally, was in another room on a table surrounded by a group of doctors and researchers.

There is now hope that the lay person can be trained to duplicate the feats formerly reserved for yogis. In biofeedback training the subject is wired to an electronic device that monitors body processes and advises him of functional activity via signals. The subject then tries to concentrate on and control, say, the blood pressure, and the machine tells him if he is succeeding.

In addition to the medical profession, promoters of conventional physical-fitness regimes are beginning to realize that mind and body are actually inseparable. At least this is the conclusion arrived at by a Purdue University physical-education professor, A. H. Ismail, who conducted a four-month test on Purdue faculty men in the thirty-to-sixty-five age range, the results of which were announced in the spring of 1972.

The experiment revealed that well-conditioned men have much more emotional stability and self-confidence than their flabby contemporaries. The correlation between physical activity and emotional health, Ismail feels, "is that middle-aged men in high-pressure, sedentary jobs develop biochemical and neurological imbalances in their body and parts of the brain. These imbalances, in turn, cause the men to become highly nervous and irritable. Physical exercise allows them to burn off these chemical and biological imbalances so that they become calm and serene."

This may be news in some circles, but it's been a fact of yoga life for four thousand years.

Belief

Belief is a key factor in yoga, and you'll be asked to believe a lot of things that can't be seen or proved scientifically. This will be easier if you realize that even in this scientific century no one has ever seen the wind, and love is yet to be duplicated in the laboratory, although the effects of both are much in evidence.

Of paramount importance in yoga is belief in yourself as a uniquely special part of the universe, belief in the human body as the most efficient machine ever designed, and a firm belief in the power of the mind.

Mind is all-important in yoga. In calisthenics rapid exercise repetitions are performed while the mind wanders. In yoga the mind must concentrate on each slow rhythmic posture and its benefits. This concentration is a form of mental discipline you can apply to all phases of your life.

Concentration

Concentration isn't an automatic ability, but it can be cultivated. The mental process of the average person resembles a shotgun blast, with thoughts going out in all directions. Concentrated thought, on the other hand, is more like a rifle shot, which goes in one direction straight toward the target. In yoga we know that concentration is controlled by controlling the way we breathe.

Yoga Breathing and Diet

When you're angry, nervous, or upset, your breathing becomes irregular and broken. When your mind and emotions calm down, the breathing again becomes calm and regular. Yoga breathing, which utilizes the full lung capacity, is a powerful tranquilizer without any bad side effects. The lung is divided into three sections, but the average person uses only the upper third section. Those doing manual labor use the upper and middle sections, and athletes, musicians, women trained for natural childbirth, and those practicing yoga breathing activate the entire lung structure.

The exhalation process is considered more important than inhalation because this is the process that rids the lungs of accumulated impurities. Antismoking and drug-abuse clinics make use of yoga breathing techniques, though not always calling it yoga. The Integral Yoga Head Program ("head" is slang for drug users) employs yoga to help addicts kick the drug habit and is supported by the New York Addiction Services

Agency. Similar programs are starting up around the country as part of the National Community Health Services Program.

Traditional yoga diet is strictly vegetarian. Worship of the sacred cow, the extremely hot Indian climate, and lack of refrigeration were undoubtedly factors favoring vegetarianism when yoga originated about 2000 B.C. Yoga purists still adhere to this vegetarian regimen, but most American yoga instructors advocate a balanced diet, with emphasis on natural foods and those not overly processed or refined.

More advanced yoga students report definite changes in their attitudes toward food, a sense of detachment about it, and a real preference for wholesome food. Moderate use of alcohol, particularly wine, is permitted, but tobacco is out.

What Yoga Will Do for You

One of yoga's greatest selling features is that it can literally "freeze one's age." The legendary Fountain of Youth has beckoned enticingly—and elusively—since its first mention in Hindu writings in the sixth century. Twentieth-century Ponce de Leons are convinced they have found it through yoga. And with half our population under twenty-eight, those over that age need all the help they can get in coping with our youth-geared society.

And there is more. An explanation of all that yoga can do for you sounds like a full-blown credibility gap. The benefits promised seem so fantastic that this form of physical fitness must be experienced to be believed. Besides reversing the aging process, yoga can eliminate tension, reduce weight, rejuvenate flagging sexual performance, instill self-confidence, completely resculpture your body, erase facial wrinkles, improve your memory by increasing circulation to the brain, lead the way toward peace of mind, and make you want to be a better human being.

Yoga also instills hope. You're never too old, too flabby, or too tense to be helped. And in our increasingly competitive society it is completely noncompetitive. Instant perfection isn't necessary, since results stem from the effort of trying to do the postures correctly. Slow and steady progress is the goal.

You don't have to be on the chill side of thirty to appreciate yoga, but it probably helps. Until then, being "over the hill" physically is something that happens to other people. Each person has two ages—numerical age and physiological age. Numerical age indicates the number of years since birth, whereas physiological age reflects the condition and appearance of the body. Numerical age can't be changed, but physiological age can be reversed by serious yoga practice.

Aging is a fact of life, and in order to combat it, we must know why people age. Time is generally considered the prime destroyer, but it is only one of many factors. Others are chronic neglect and exhaustion, improper diet, stress, insufficient exercise, and lack of mental interests. But the most powerful enemies of youth and attractiveness are the pull of central gravity and decreasing blood circulation in the face and head. These two work hand in hand, and the same gravitational pull that keeps you "down to earth" is also responsible for sagging muscles, displaced organs, fallen arches, and the inclination to sit or lie down rather than stand up.

Yoga's remedy for this is simple and sensible—the body is turned upside down. With gravity's pull reversed, those dragged-down muscles and organs are now pulled in the opposite way and restored to their original and proper positions. These inverted postures also provide an increased flow of blood to the face and head and feed sagging and starved facial tissues. The entire system—glands, organs, and nerve roots—is revitalized by the extra supply of arterial blood.

Critics of yoga claim that it creates an unhealthy interest in the physical body. Despite the fact that one is considered legally of age at twenty-one, in yoga it is felt that emotional maturity is not reached until about age forty-five. By this time the body is often pretty much past its prime—the forties in this country bring on heart attacks, obesity, and ulcers. Through yoga, one should be able to remain forty-five physically for perhaps as long as thirty years, being comfortable with the body, able to enjoy the maturity at long last achieved.

Legend has it that Patanjali, called the father of yoga, went into the mountains, meditated, and emerged to write the system that is now known as yoga. The fact is that Patanjali was a man of mystery about whom little is known. Scholars are even at odds as to when he lived and worked, their guesses ranging from the fourth century B.C. to the fourth century A.D. The most commonly accepted date is the second century B.C.

Patanjali did not originate yoga—its doctrine has been handed down from prehistoric times—but he collected the findings, knowledge, and opinions of other yogis and aligned them with his own experiences. He then restated the yoga philosophy in definite principles and precise teachings in a work formally titled *Aphorisms on Yoga*, or *Yoga Sutras*,* a treatise on raja-yoga.

* The word *sutra* means thread, and Patanjali's writings were the threads of ideas, mere skeletal outlines intended for the use of teachers who would verbally expand and explain them. Although the sutras are extremely difficult to follow and understand, their terse style was justified, as they were composed at a time when there were no books. The entire work was memorized and handed down through the ages.

Branches of Yoga

The wise men of the East who originated yoga knew that no one system for reaching God would appeal to all people. There are, therefore, five main branches of yoga—karma-yoga, bhaki-yoga, jnana-yoga, hatha-yoga, and raja-yoga—and each has its own appeal, depending on the seeker's basic interests and personality.

Karma-yoga is the spiritual path characterized by right action and service to others. Karma is a familiar word to believers in reincarnation, those who feel that a soul returns to earth many times to learn various spiritual lessons. This subject will be covered in a separate chapter, but "karma" means cause and effect, or action and reaction, and can be compared to the biblical "as ye sow, so shall ye reap," and "an eye for an eye, a tooth for a tooth."

Those who mistreat others—by thought, word, or deed—will receive the same kind of treatment in return in this life or the next. Lives that epitomize the Golden Rule, "do unto others as you would have them do unto you," are lives lived in accordance with karma-yoga, whether it is called that or not. A life spent doing the right thing and helping others without concern for personal gain or reward builds "good karma" to offset past human errors. These soul debits help equalize one's total karma, which could be called the "balance sheet of the soul."

Bhakti-yoga is the path of spiritual enlightenment through worship and devotion to the Supreme Being, essentially the path of the monk, priest, or nun.

Jnana-yoga is the intellectual path to self-realization and union with God through knowledge and wisdom. Many of our early literary figures, including Emerson, Thoreau, and Whitman, initially espoused this route to universal truth. Their quests were so deep and consuming that they ultimately progressed to raja-yoga, the kingly yoga.

Hatha-yoga, the primary subject of this book, is the path to God through complete mental and physical control. In its advanced stages hatha-yoga merges wtih raja-yoga. The primary authoritative text for this branch is the *Hatha Yoga Pradipika*, by Svatmarama, who is known as the codifier of hatha-yoga.

Raja-yoga is the highest form of yoga, the royal union with the Universal Spirit through meditation. A raja-yogi is one who has complete mastery over the self, one who has conquered his body, mind, senses, passions, and thoughts and is a king among men.

India: Mother of Yoga

All yoga originated in India, a poverty-ridden country one-third the geographical size of the United States. Approximately one of every seven persons in the world lives in India, where there are 396 persons per square mile, compared to 54 per square mile in the United States. Although there are some wealthy Indians, the average income is seventy-eight dollars per year. Many Indians live on five cents or less a day and consider themselves blessed if they have food to stay alive and shelter for sleeping at night.

Despite the numbing poverty that now grips this country, India was not always a destitute nation. It was, in fact, the wealthiest country in the world until the eighteenth century. Indian history dates back at least 4,500 years, and archaeological excavations at Mohenjo-daro and Harrappa (now in Pakistan) reveal the existence of an advanced civilization in the Indus Valley as long ago as 3000 B.C. These ruins indicate a culture that had many conveniences not found in most Indian villages today, where inhabitants lived in multistoried brick homes arranged along well-planned streets that formed city blocks. These people had their own wells, bathrooms, sewer systems, and large public baths as well as handsome jewelry, well-made household utensils, and copper weapons. This advanced civilization, which also had a system of counting, measuring, weighing, and writing, disappeared without a trace. No one knows what happened to the people.

The India that once symbolized wealth, mystery, culture, and excitement to the Western world has been eroded throughout history by alien invasion, religious wars, and a rapidly burgeoning population until now its only world legacy is its spiritual knowledge. In fact, the masters who have emerged in every generation are India's truest wealth.

Spiritual Supermen

A look at the masters of India is a mind-boggling experience for most Westerners. These miracle men of the East exhibit powers that, from Christianity's viewpoint, were possible only for Jesus Christ. Christianity's reverence for Christ is shared by the Hindus, although they do not regard Him as the only son of God, but one of many sons, along with Buddha, Krishna, and others.

For a fully illumined master, all things are possible. Their miracles include healing the sick, raising the dead, complete knowledge of past, present, and future, clairvoyance, clairaudience, telepathy, and physical bilocation—the power to materialize an additional body in another location when necessary. But more about this in a later chapter.

An avatar is a god descended to earth in human form, and though India's history abounds with them, their existence has created barely a ripple in Western awareness where material giants command more respect than spiritual ones. However, in the early years of the 1970s, even the Western world is taking note of Indian avatar Sai Baba, a seemingly incredible man who is said to heal the sick and produce fruit, flowers, sweets, jewels, and sacred ashes (*vibhuti*) with a mere wave of his hand.

Satyanarayana was born November 23, 1926, in a remote Indian village. On the eve of his birth it is said that musical instruments in the family hut played melodiously without human assistance. He displayed unusual powers even as a child, and at the age of fourteen announced to his family that he was the reincarnation of Sai Baba, the Saint of Shirdi. The original Sai Baba died in 1918, vowing to his disciples that he would again take earthly form in eight years. Many of the original Baba's disciples are still living and are convinced that their master lives again.

The current Sai Baba materializes objects, is impervious to pain, and displays such supernormal abilities as precognition, telepathy, and physical bilocation. His devotees believe that these powers are meant to teach man that our next great step in evolutionary growth will be from a mental to a supermental state of being. While miracles of the magnitude produced by Sai Baba are hard for the materially geared mind to grasp, his detractors find it hard to explain his motivation, since he accepts no money or gifts from his followers. One of his most ardent devotees is Indra Devi, noted teacher of yoga and author of several books on the subject.

A California businessman became curious about Sai Baba after hearing of his exploits from Mataji,* Indra Devi is affectionately called in India and also by her Western followers. She tells this story: On a subsequent trip to India, he and a group of Californians met Sai Baba and witnessed his miracles. They were all still skeptical, and asked India's reigning miracle man to show further proof of his divinity. The group was speechless when Sai Baba "took from the air" a rosary of twenty-one pearls, which he gave to Indra Devi, after endowing it with healing properties.

Another skeptic turned devotee is Dr. S. Bhagavantam, a top Indian scientist, who visited Sai Baba, but clearly doubted the swami's abilities. Sai Baba took his visitor for a walk along the river in the village, and in the course of the conversation asked him whether, as a scientist, he believed in the *Bhagavad-Gita* (the Hindu bible), and whether he would like a copy of it.

---

* *Mataji*, in Sanskrit, means Holy Mother. The suffix, *ji*, is a term of endearment that is often given a guru by his disciples, as "Swamiji."

"Yes, and I would cherish a copy of it," Bhagavatam replied.

Sai Baba knelt down and with cupped hands scooped some sand into a small mound. He then picked up the mound, and as he did so, the sand was transformed into a beautifully bound copy of the sacred book. The astonished, but still pragmatic, scientist immediately turned to the front of the book in search of the publisher's name. There was none.

"Sai Press," the miracle man said, smiling.

2

THE IMPORTANCE
OF ATTITUDES

When John Kemp was born without arms or legs, a doctor advised his parents to take their tiny son home, place him in a basket, and make him as comfortable as possible for the rest of his life. Fortunately, his parents ignored this bit of negative advice, and because they did, John Kemp has accomplished more in twenty-three years than many of his peers.

Despite gross physical abnormalities, John Kemp is more fortunate than countless "normal" people because he was born into a family in which positive mental attitudes were a way of life. Johnny's mother died of cancer when he was fifteen months old, leaving his father, John B. Kemp, to raise the boy and his three-month- and five-year-old sisters. The prime mover in the success story of this young man is his father, who convinced him that despite being a congenital quadruple amputee, he was not handicapped.

Limitation Is a Mental Thing

John Kemp is *not* handicapped. He's probably one of the most normal people around. Fitted with artificial arms at age two and artificial legs at three, he candidly admits that "I am convinced there are no absolute limits to my abilities." One of the biggest hang-ups in personal achievement is that so many people are conditioned to accept the idea of limitation, and limitation originates entirely in the mind—either your own or that of someone who has had an influence over you.

The best-seller *Jonathan Livingston Seagull* deals with the theory of limitation, urges us to disregard it, and states allegorically that "you are, from wingtip to wingtip, pure thought." For those who haven't read this excellent book, may I translate: Do not accept anyone else's idea of what you can do—anything you *believe* you can achieve, you *can* achieve.

While the upper limits of our abilities in many fields are determined by our genetic inheritance, few of us ever come even remotely close to scaling our personal mountaintops. Young John Kemp loved sports, particularly baseball, and learned early to throw a great fast ball and to be a first-rate fly-catcher. He was so convinced that limitation is mental that his father's most difficult task was convincing him that a career in big-league baseball was not in the cards.

"Each of us has unique abilities," his wise father counseled, "and you must learn to use your head instead of your body to succeed in this life."

John uses his head well. A graduate of Georgetown University, he attends law school at Washburn University where academic life is well balanced by an active dating and social life. He held class offices in both high school and college and earned a 90.2 academic average in high school, along with seven varsity letters as student manager of the basketball, track, and swimming teams. Sound normal?

"You are what you think," John says, "and in day-to-day living, I was never regarded as handicapped, and thus I have never felt that I am."

Besides his head, John uses his gift of humor, his charismatic good looks, and a great amount of heart to help those he feels are less fortunate than he. Having been named the National Easter Seal Child in 1960, he now serves as the youngest board member in the fifty-four-year history of the National Easter Seal Society, has served on the President's Committee on Employment of the Handicapped, and is currently active in a project to galvanize the youth of the nation to help the handicapped.

Difference between the Optimist and the Pessimist Is Attitude

John Kemp is a perfect example of the difference between an optimist and a pessimist. There is an old cliché that aptly defines this difference: The optimist says we live in the best of all possible worlds; the pessimist fears this is true. The basic difference, then, between an optimist and a pessimist is attitude. Defining intangibles—and attitudes are intangible—produces a glazed look in many eyes. The dictionary defines an attitude as a way of thinking, acting, or feeling. Going a step further, attitudes are positive or negative, good or bad.

Attitudes being intangible, you can't see one or touch one, but the results of attitudes are totally tangible and concrete. We live in a world of cause and effect, and our lives are the direct result of our attitudes. Even though attitudes are not visible to the naked eye, walk down any street and you will see the results of attitudes clearly etched on the faces you pass, because outer countenance and facial expression reflect the inner self— one's attitudes. The man with ugly downward lines in his expression is negative inside, just as a tightly pinched mouth and rigid facial set inadequately mask the woman whose interests do not extend beyond herself. To the discerning eye, the inner you is inerasably imprinted on the face you present to the world.

The role our attitudes play in determining whether we have a happy or unhappy life is dramatically demonstrated by many married couples who, though living basically the same life, see it differently due to differing attitudes. Bob and Betty M. have a comfortable income, with Bob securely employed in the field of his choice, own their own home, and are the parents of two healthy, bright, talented, and beautiful children. This couple would seem to represent the American dream, but unfortunately, because of incompatible attitudes, this potentially idyllic situation leaves much to be desired.

One need not be a psychologist to detect the problem of this marriage. Bob's facial expression is unfailingly a pleasant one; to one and all he is courteous, cheerful, and optimistic. Betty's face is a study in anger, dissatisfaction, and frustration. Even though Bob loves his job, Betty finds reasons for resenting her husband's boss and his working conditions; the house that was built to her specifications doesn't suit her; she never has enough money to spend; and the personalities and activities of her children provide a fertile field for her omnipresent irritation. Regardless of what her life situation had been, this woman would always have been unhappy. She's incapable of happiness because of her attitudes. Unfortunately, she will probably never realize that her unhappiness is all of her own making.

Take a moment now to objectively observe the attitudes represented on your face. Look in the mirror, and without rearranging your features for public view, really examine what is there. Emerson once observed: "That only which we have within, can we see without. If we meet no gods, it is because we harbor none."

Since man first stood upright and pondered his nature there have been a few enlightened individuals who realized that they themselves ruled their destinies. The *Yoga Sutras* establish that human unhappiness results when man accepts and is subservient to the improper condition of his own mind.

In other words, "As a man thinketh, so is he." Followers of the sutras, and of all branches of yoga, are shown how to overcome improper thinking and progress toward health, beauty, peace, prosperity, and all the worthwhile things of this world.

The biblical aphorism "As a man thinketh in his heart, so is he," from Proverbs, has served as a catalyst for inspirational writings for centuries. James Allen's classic volume *As a Man Thinketh* states that man's thinking "not only embraces the whole of a man's being, but is so comprehensive as to reach out to every condition and circumstance of his life. A man is literally what he thinks, his character being the complete sum of all his thoughts."

Allen's thinking parallels yogic belief—that the law of cause and effect is as absolute and undeviating in the hidden realm of thought as in the world of visible and material things. Every experience, even the so-called spontaneous or unpremeditated one, is the effect—the end result—that has been created and caused by the power of thought. Good and noble human beings don't just happen by accident; they are created by good and noble thoughts, just as reprehensible characters are created by ugly and negative thoughts.

Your Physical Body Is the Result of Your Thoughts

One's character is not the only result of one's thinking; the physical body is also created along the trails and footpaths of the mind. Yoga literature presents an illustration of the mind's power to resculpture the body in the story of the Tiger Swami, the Hindu equivalent of Charles Atlas.

Born with a burning desire to fight tigers, coupled with the body of a ninety-seven-pound weakling, the Tiger Swami seemed destined for failure. After his prowess in manually subduing the fierce Bengal tigers had spread throughout India, and after he had turned his hand to the taming of spiritual tigers instead of jungle ones, he told the story of his physical transformation.

> Mind is the wielder of muscles. The force of a hammer blow depends on the energy applied; the power expressed by a man's bodily instrument depends on his aggressive will and courage. The body is literally manufactured and sustained by mind. Through pressure of instincts from past lives, strengths or weaknesses percolate gradually into human consciousness. They express as habits, which in turn manifest as a desirable or an undesirable body. Outward frailty has a mental origin; in a vicious circle, the habit-bound body thwarts the mind. If the master allows himself to be commanded by a servant, the latter becomes autocratic; the mind is similarly enslaved by submitting to bodily dictation.

The Power of Positive Thinking

The importance of attitudes, particularly the power of positive ones, can't be stressed too strongly, although that isn't the primary purpose of this book. I have touched on attitudes because they are an integral part of the physical, mental, and spiritual developmental system that is yoga. And your success in yoga will be determined largely by your attitudes.

For an in-depth study of thought power, may I recommend Norman Vincent Peale's *The Power of Positive Thinking*, an all-time best-seller and a classic in its field. If you've already read it, read it again. For those who want a how-to-do-it book for applying positive attitudes to the business of business, Napoleon Hill's *Think and Grow Rich* and *Grow Rich with Peace of Mind* rank at the top, and they are worthwhile even if your goals are not material ones. If your interests are along spiritual lines, don't let the implication of these titles mislead you—they're not geared to the fast-buck artist, but refer to a richness of life that can be applied to all facets of existence. Also on the recommended reading list is *Success through a Positive Mental Attitude*, by Napoleon Hill and W. Clement Stone.

Have you ever wondered about the genesis of those attitudes and thought patterns that make you the person you are? Eric Berne, of *Games People Play* fame, wrote a book, published posthumously, entitled *What Do You Say after You Say Hello?*, which explains the origin of our attitudes and self-image. This book, along with *I'm OK, You're OK*, by Thomas A. Harris, should be required reading for anyone interested in self-knowledge.

In the vernacular of our electronic age your attitudes are the result of programming—programming that has been going on since the day you were born. The first time your mother looked into your baby-blue eyes, whether in adoration, awe, resentment, or disappointment, she was setting in motion the image you have of yourself today and the attitudes you have toward the world. Each subsequent encounter with parents, siblings, and the outside world further enlarged, decreased, or altered your self-image and, correspondingly, your attitudes.

The Catholic Church has long known the impact of early programming, and their belief that given a child up to the age of six, he will be theirs for life is well founded. Scientists, in their recent studies of brain-wave activity, have reached the conclusion that attitudes and thinking patterns that are imbedded in the mind during the plastic years of early childhood remain even though they are contradictory to the intellect and reason that develop later in life. In other words, your conscious mind and intelligence may tell you that race is no barometer of athletic ability, but if early programming implanted the notion that the Negro race produces better athletes, that notion will stick. This is the same reason that old wives' tales, many of which have no basis in fact, are perpetrated from generation to generation.

From Beta to Delta and Back Again

Alphagenics, the study of human brain-wave activity, may be the science of the 1970s that will break the death grip the mind has on the physical body. It may revolutionize our concepts about our own abilities, make us individually responsible for our attitudes, and necessitate a complete restructuring of the medical profession as well as psychiatry.

There are four known levels of brain-wave frequency: beta, alpha, theta, and delta. Beta, which ranges from 14 to 55 cycles per second, is the brain-wave frequency associated with the five known physical senses of sight, hearing, taste, touch, and smell. This is the outer conscious level, at which we function during our normal everyday activities.

Alpha, with brain-wave frequencies from 7 to 14 cycles per second, is an inner conscious level associated with the dream state, extrasensory perception, creative visualization, complete relaxation, and meditation. This frequency is also associated with accelerated healing, with 10½ cycles per second thought to be optimum.

Theta, from 4 to 7 cycles per second, is the brain-wave frequency prevailing in hypnosis and anesthesia, and in delta, from 0 to 4 cycles per second, one is in deep sleep or unconscious.

The normal brain cycles through all levels constantly, but the average adult spends 80 percent of waking time in beta. The intoxicated person cycles uncontrollably from a high beta through alpha; marijuana produces an alpha trip, although cigarette smoking depresses the alpha function; and with LSD there is cycling through all levels.

Brain-wave activity is also related to a person's age. The infant, from birth to age four, spends most of its existence in theta and delta, the levels of hypnosis and deep sleep; four-to-seven-year-olds produce a preponderance of theta waves, the level of hypnosis; from seven to fourteen, 55 percent of the time is spent at the lower brain levels, mostly alpha. From the age of fourteen through the remainder of life, the average person's brain-wave activity is predominantly beta.

Why Early Programming Sticks

Beta relates to the conscious objective mind, and the lower levels correspond to the subconscious or subjective levels of mind. Since children spend more than 50 percent of their time at lower brain frequency levels, information impressed upon them is rooted in the subconscious where it sticks. An adult under hypnosis, the theta level, can be given a post-hypnotic suggestion that at the stroke of 8:00 P.M. he will become uncomfortably cold. And at 8:00 P.M. the thermometer may register 90°, but the subject's subconscious will overrule his conscious intellect, and he will shiver in spite of his overcoat.

Children are much like the adult under hypnosis, and their early programming, whether positive or negative, like a posthypnotic suggestion, will be reflected in attitudes and behavior the rest of their lives. Compounding this problem is the fact that children have no corrective information to offset negative programming.

Verbal and Nonverbal Programming

Paul's earliest memories are of his mother's warnings: "Don't run. You'll fall down and hurt yourself." Later, it was, "If you play with the hammer, you're going to smash your fingers." During grade school the theme was, "Don't ride your bike in the street because of the cars," and in high school, "Playing football is a good way to get your teeth knocked out." Today her son is grown, and this mother can't understand why her fear-ridden offspring is a misfit in the world of men.

Destructive as this type of programming is, being verbal, it is out in the open for scrutiny should Paul decide to reprogram himself and scale down his fears, restructuring his life in a more realistic manner. How this can be accomplished is explained later in this chapter.

There are more subtle types of programming that are more insidious because they are nonverbal; in fact, frequently the words that accompany this programming are in direct contradiction to the actual programming. This programming involves verbalization plus body language, which is less subject to self-deception.

Examples of this kind of programming abound in parent-child relationships. Mothers, most of whom have been instilled with the notion that motherhood is next to sainthood, often find in reality that they resent the demands children make on their time and the sacrifices expected of them. This pull between the mother's early programming and her own interests now shows up in her relationship with her children, though she is often unaware of it.

In this situation the mother may verbally tell her child that he's the most important thing in her life, while she is literally holding the child at arm's length. Children read body language easily, and the implications of such a transaction are not lost on them. This translates to the child that while mother says he's lovable and important, she shows by her actions that she doesn't really mean it.

The most insidious and the most subtle programming of all is nonverbal and does not employ body language. It is telepathic, strictly mind-to-mind programming. Kids are naturally intuitive, existing as they do in an alpha-theta world of brain-wave activity, and they "pick up" many of the thoughts of those around them without the thinker being aware of it.

My younger child, who was born in 1967, is a constant reminder of the actuality of thought transference. The following examples are typical.

Our family menagerie includes a couple of cats that greet each new day with ravenous appetites, and as any cat owner knows, it's very diffi-cult to ignore a hungry cat. One morning our dog, in a fit of animal sibling rivalry, ate the last can of cat food, and I was considering placating the unhappy cats with a can of tuna. Although I did not mention this, my then five-year-old daughter, Page, said, "I don't think you should do that."

"Do what?" I asked.

"I don't think you should feed tuna to the cats, because it's too expen-sive," she replied matter-of-factly.

Swami Rama tells me this child was a yogi in another life, so maybe she isn't typical, but another example of her telepathic knowledge is even stranger. A rainy spring Sunday had reduced our yard to the consistency of a swamp, and both my children kept bringing groups of neighbor children into the house. After one of their trips inside, while I was cleaning the front hall for the fourth time that day, I thought, "I'd like to put a great big sign on that front door saying KEEP OUT."

Page came inside alone and was playing quietly in her room when my older daughter, Robin, and the peanut-butter set again traipsed through the front hall. Page called to her sister, "What's the matter with you, Robin? Can't you see that sign on the front door?"

"What are you talking about?" Robin asked.

"There's a big sign on the front door that says KEEP OUT." Page's answer implied that her older sister's senses were faulty.

Robin assured Page that there was no sign on the door, and, of course, there wasn't one. At the time the thought of a sign crossed my mind, Page was outside, and I had not mentioned the thought to her. But the strangest thing of all is that had there been a sign on the door, Page, at age five, couldn't have read it!

My children routinely tune in to what I'm thinking of preparing for dinner, what I'm planning to wear on any given occasion, and send me mental requests to pick them up when the distance home from a friend's house looks discouragingly long from the viewpoint of a tired youngster. They are amused if I think picking them up was my idea. Of course, both of them have been trained to use mind power from early childhood, and they're not above using it to jog my maternal instincts.

These are harmless examples of totally mental programming, but this same faculty is activated destructively when a mother or anyone else who is around a child allows his or her mind to dwell on negative thoughts about the child. Thinking that a child is a nuisance, or stupid, or unattractive, or not as lovable as a sibling is lowering that child's self-esteem just as surely as if you had verbalized these feelings.

Alexander Smith, author of *On the Importance of a Man to Himself*, showed knowledge of the power of attitudes and programming when he stated, "In the wide arena of the world, failure and success are not accidents as we so frequently suppose, but the strictest justice." The "losers" in life's battle are the ones whose parents inadvertently programmed them for failures with comments such as, "You're never going to amount to anything," "It's always the rich kids who get the good grades," and "You're not smart enough to make the honor roll." And the success stories of life didn't just happen either, but were positively programmed with, "We know you have the intelligence to make the honor roll—just apply yourself," and other positive suggestions that produced the end result of success.

Faith, hope, optimism, and compassion are all instilled attitudes, just as are fear, negativity, and bigotry. Anyone who has watched television's *All in the Family* will recognize Archie Bunker as the epitome of prejudiced and bigoted programming. Presented in the form of entertainment, the juxtaposition of Archie's immature and negative personality to that of his liberal and positively programmed daughter and son-in-law brings attitudes to life.

Programming Can Be Changed

Are you hamstrung by your attitudes? Does your early programming weigh around your neck like the Ancient Mariner's albatross, pigeonholing you in the slot of an also-ran? If you recognize this as your problem, be thankful, because recognition of the problem is the first step in its solution. Start by seeing your situation from the standpoint of an optimist: The more negative you are now and the more unsatisfactory your life situation, the greater and more dramatic will be the changes created by altering your inner structure.

"That's a bunch of pollyanna nonsense" is the standard reaction of the negative thinker. To this, and every other negative thought or statement, mentally or aloud say "cancel-cancel," a technique developed by José Silva, founder of Silva Mind Control, which is explained later in this chapter. Pseudosophistication and objective thinking to the contrary, in reprogramming your subconscious you must resort to seemingly childlike phrases, and you must have the faith of a child.

Reprogramming is really retraining your subconscious. Visualize your subconscious as the genie of the lamp—huge, all-powerful, all-knowing, the custodian of your every thought and action. This omnipresent giant never sleeps, regulates the functioning of all automatic bodily functions, always knows what time it is without resorting to clocks, and remembers exactly what you were doing ten years ago last Thursday—but it doesn't have a sense of humor.

This tremendously impressive creation is your own personal slave, but it is a very literal one. Directed entirely by your thoughts and spoken words, it will produce exactly what you think and say. If you say one thing, in an effort to impress someone or because it is the thing to do but really think otherwise, your subconscious follows the dictates of your real thought. Like a mechanical robot, the subconscious has no sense of right or wrong and depends on you as its master for correct instructions.

When you say, "My husband gives me a pain in the neck," your subconscious produces what you have requested. When you think, "I'll never land that job," your subconscious will lead you into situations and actions to make sure you don't land the job. And when a momentary lapse of memory occurs, a comment such as, "I can't remember, I'll probably think of it at three o'clock in the morning," translates to your subconscious, the storehouse of all memory, as, "Don't drag it out now, he really wants this information in the middle of the night."

Keep Your Vocabulary Positive

Step one in reprogramming your attitudes, and your life, is reprogramming your vocabulary. Even though this may seem silly at first, and even though you don't really think it will help, start immediately to eliminate statements such as:

"I'll never amount to anything. . . ."
"I'll never really be healthy. . . ."
"I'll never have enough time. . . ."
"I'll never be able to do the Headstand. . . ."
"I'll never be able to stop smoking. . . ."
"I'll never be able to lose this weight. . . ."
"I'll never have any self-confidence. . . ."
"My kids are driving me crazy. . . ."

If you slip and make a negative statement, or even think negatively, invoke the magic of "cancel-cancel," a note to the subconscious to strike that from the record.

Visualize the Desired End Result

Step two in reprogramming is to visualize the desired end result. Problems are so universal that life could be called a series of problems to be solved. When confronted with a problem that needs a solution, consider all the phases of it that are known to you, and determine what it is that you want to happen.

From that point on, don't keep rehashing the elements of the problem—keep your mind focused on the desired end result. See, in your mind's eye, the problem as solved. Don't concern yourself with the details of the solution; these will be provided by your all-powerful subconscious, which is not limited by the logic of the objective mind.

If the problem is a financial one, mentally "see" your bank statement showing the exact sum you need to accomplish your goal. If your heart is set on finding your personal dream home, visualize it, mentally stroll through its rooms, and see yourself living there. If you wish to lose weight, see yourself thin instead of dwelling on those extra pounds.

The ability to visualize, to form specific mental images at will, is a valuable fringe benefit of yoga. In attempting a difficult posture, it is important to your ultimate success that you be able to mentally see yourself performing it correctly. And visualization is equally important in anything else you are trying to accomplish because it is a creative function: To visualize is to create—mentally. That which you can see clearly in your mind's eye you can actually produce.

The genius of Albert Einstein may have resulted from his "extraordinary capacity for nonverbal communication"—in other words, visualization. Unable or unwilling to speak until the age of three, he later said: "I rarely think in words at all. A thought comes, and I may try to express it in words afterward."

Yoga is a tool for living, and its disciplines and techniques should be integrated into the business of life. Some people have trouble learning to visualize, but this ability improves with practice. Start simply by closing your eyes and mentally picturing your car, home, relatives, and pets. Expand these practice sessions by taking a mental walk around an area that you know well. Soon you will find yourself seeing with your mind's eye automatically.

Affirmations

An affirmation is a positive statement, an assertion of fact, and is the third reprogramming tool. The title of Sammy Davis, Jr.'s, book, *Yes, I Can,* is an affirmation, as is his life. One of Christianity's most powerful affirmations is the 23rd Psalm, which is a masterful example of the correct use of an affirmation; namely, it is stated in the present tense and as though the desired end result were already an accomplished fact. Present-tense phrasing is imperative.

When you say, "I am going to lose weight," your all-literal, nonhumorous subconscious translates thusly: "Don't shed the weight now—she's going to lose it later." Anytime you use an affirmation in the future tense, your subconscious will not produce it for you now. Use the present tense always: I am thin, I am healthy, I am successful. . . .

Develop your own affirmation, stating as accomplished fact whatever you wish to happen. Write it down, memorize it, and say it to yourself, aloud or mentally, several times each day. With each repetition the affirmation grows stronger in your subconscious.

There are spiritual laws governing the subtle realms of existence that are just as precise and exacting as those that govern the physical universe. Ignorance of the law of gravity is no protection should one leap from a skyscraper, and the misuse of spiritual laws governing the power of the mind can be equally devastating. Krishnamurti, one of this century's greatest teachers and writers, once said, "Be careful of what you wish—you may get it." Far from being an attempt at humor, this statement reveals a real understanding of the power of thought.

Concentration: the Passive Power That Makes It Work

The fourth and final step in reprogramming is concentration, defined in Patanjali's *Aphorisms on Yoga* as "holding the mind steadily fixed on some particular object." Each of us has been told since childhood to concentrate, to keep your mind on what you are doing, to "put your mind to it." Concentration is something most Westerners find difficult, because our lives and our culture are filled with such a multitude of distractions, not the least of which are radio, television, and the telephone. Another reason it is difficult is that we have never been taught how to concentrate.

Even very small children can be taught the fine art of concentration while helping with household chores. For example, little girls helping clean up the kitchen after meals should be taught to start at one given spot and clear and clean each counter surface before going to the next area. By working counterclockwise and completely finishing one area before going on to the next area, they will be learning efficient homemaking and concentration at the same time.

Counting sheep to induce sleep is a form of concentration. By visualizing sheep jumping over a fence and counting them, the mind is closed to outside distractions. Another aid to concentration is rhythmic breathing, which will be outlined in the next chapter.

Yoga teaches the use of the mind for meditation, for creative visualization, and for concentration. Of the three, concentration is probably the most difficult to master, because it means to hold the mind on one specific subject for lengthening periods of time.

In meditation man quiets his conscious mind so that in the silence he will be able to tune in to Higher Consciousness for knowledge, for the correct solution to a problem. With the creative force, visualization, he forms a mental picture of that solution. And with concentration he provides energy or power to achieve the desired solution. The longer he can hold his concentration on that which he has visualized, the quicker it will come to pass in actuality.

Many of the postures in yoga are so complicated, so involved, that they seem ridiculous. While they all have profound physical benefits, the main reason for their complexity is that doing the unusual requires concentration, but the more one uses concentration, the easier it becomes.

Let's Reprogram

Set aside five minutes a day to start reprogramming; they can be the last five minutes of your waking day, just before you go to sleep. Close your eyes, relax your body, and breathe deeply and rhythmically; this will lower your brain-wave frequency so that subconscious impressions will be imprinted more strongly. Repeat your affirmation mentally, and at the same time see your goal as accomplished in your mind's eye. Don't let your mind wander. Keep repeating your affirmation mentally. Thought has power, and the more concentrated it is, the more power it has. Our most concentrated thought centers on that which we desire most.

A case in point is that of Marie M., a beautiful blonde who ardently desired a husband—not just any husband, but a very specific one. Her list of specifications was long and precise. Utilizing the affirmation technique, coupled with visualization, she set aside three or four periods during each day for concentrating on the husband of her choice. Reared in Europe, she desired a husband with sufficient time and income to allow them to spend a month each year in Europe. She had decided that he must be tall and slim and distinguished-looking, with a moustache and goatee, and that he must also share her enthusiasms for tennis, people, reading, travel, and the color pink. Since she is unable to have children, he must have had children by a previous marriage. Her requirements were endlessly detailed, topped by her most important requirement—he must absolutely adore her!

What were the results of her mental programming? Well, for the past two years Marie has been happily married to a tall, slim, distinguished-looking stockbroker with moustache and goatee. They go to Europe for a month each year, socialize a great deal, play a lot of tennis, and so on through Marie's entire list. She and her friends teasingly suggest that he is a figment of her imagination, that she actually conjured up this dream marriage in her mind. Strange as this sounds, it's a perfect example of the law of attraction—that which the mind dwells on the mind attracts.

The law of attraction works on negative thoughts just as dramatically as it does on positive ones. One man, whose primary fear in life was losing his job, eventually did—through his own mental processes. Constantly dwelling on that fear provided the concentrated energy necessary to bring it into reality.

Mind Control: Ancient and Modern

One of the goals of hatha-yoga is mind control, called *dharana* in Sanskrit, and it is achieved through mental suggestion, the constant mental repetition that eventually sinks into the subconscious and becomes fact. Mind control is not the sole province of yoga, and students of the Bible will agree that many of its teachings are actually forms of mind control. But despite its fantastic potential, the mind has been largely ignored by much of the world.

There's nothing new about mind control, and you can learn to use your mind more effectively by yourself—but it does require reading, study, and practice. For those who prefer personal instruction, a system has been developed that is enjoying a great degree of success in the United States, Mexico, and Canada called Silva Mind Control.

This system, called "the beginning of the second phase of human evolution" by its proponents, is based on the concept that although the brain does not go outside the human body for information, the mind does. This system began as an experiment into how children's IQ's might be raised, and it took a surprising turn when the children in the control group began demonstrating extrasensory perception.

Another basic premise of Silva Mind Control is that ESP is not "extra" at all, but a prior sense that fell into disuse when language developed, eliminating the need for mind-to-mind contact.

Silva Mind Control, in a nutshell, is self-control of the human mind by learning to voluntarily control brain-wave frequencies, particularly the alpha wave. While this program is geared to the lay person, similar work is being done in the medical profession in biofeedback training, in which patients are taught to control heart rate, blood pressure, and other physiological processes previously considered involuntary.

The forty-eight-hour mind-control course is composed of lectures and conditioning cycles, called programming. The human mind is compared to a computer, and it is pointed out that what is programmed into the mind is projected back in behavior and attitudes that are consistent with the programming.

"Many of the problems people experience are the result of prior negative programming," a mind-control instructor points out, cautioning parents that when they tell a child he or she will never amount to anything, that parent is programming the child for failure in the future.

All forms of negative thinking and behavior are attacked in a mind-control course. It goes into the vast power of the subconscious, and students are taught that the difference between a genius mentality and a lay person's mentality is that a genius uses more of his mind and uses it in a special manner—and they are learning to use more of their mind and use it in a special manner.

The medical profession now acknowledges that upward of 50 percent of all illness is emotionally or psychologically induced, and mind-control students are programmed never to develop mentally or physically a number of man's dreaded ailments, such as arthritis, heart disease, emphysema, or cancer. Additional programming drills into students' subconscious minds that they will never be affected by their negative thoughts or those of others and that every day in every way they are getting better and better. Unsophisticated, childlike? Yes, but it's effective. It's a little Norman Vincent Peale, a little Pavlov, and a little Coué—with a José Silva twist.

A full rundown on Silva Mind Control is impossible here, but graduates report the ability to banish pain, insomnia, anxiety, and tension, improve memory and IQ, solve problems through dreams, and program success and achievement into business and personal lives. They also claim to have increased extrasensory perception and clairvoyance.

In the last class of a mind-control course students are told they will be given only the name, address, age, and sex of a person with a physical or mental problem and that the student will be able to detect the problem. Mind control boasts 100 percent success, with the proof of this success being the student's ability to do just this—"work cases."

Throughout the entire course, which contains much that is strange to the rigid thinker, students are urged to accept or reject whatever they wish. The possibility of psychic diagnosis causes many people who have accepted the program up to that point to hit the reject button. I took the course and doubted my ability to pass this required test. But I did pass, with 100 percent accuracy, in describing the physical characteristics including height, weight, skin, and hair color—and physical deformity—of a stranger. This person was not in the class with me, and the problems he had were listed on a card that I did not see.

When working cases, you sit with eyes closed and count down, as you have been taught, to the alpha level. The person holding the card containing pertinent data on the case then tells you that the individual in question "will now appear on your mental screen." To my amazement, at the proper time, I saw quite distinctly a man in his mid-twenties with dark, curly hair, who appeared about 5'10" tall and weighed approximately 165 pounds. Without my effort the young man turned so that I could see the side view of his body and a spinal deformity that I "sensed" caused pain in his left leg. Then it seemed that I was peering through this young man's eyes, and as I looked down, I noted that his left leg was encased, from ankle to hip, in a steel brace. I was recounting what I felt and saw, and the card-holder confirmed that I was totally accurate in describing his brother-in-law, whose left leg is in a brace, the aftermath of a childhood polio attack.

At the time it seemed incredible, and it still does. Mind control is both exciting and unsettling. It's exciting to realize how much more of our mind, our billion-dollar computer, we can learn to use. It's unsettling because it changes the foundation of our beliefs about ourselves and our potential—and change is always unsettling.

Those who feel that heightened awareness, such as is developed through mind control and through yoga, amounts to the usurping of powers best left to Christ can take heart from the words of Christ: "And these signs shall follow them that believe: In my name they shall cast out devils; they shall speak with new tongues; they shall take up serpents; and if they drink any deadly thing, it shall not hurt them; they shall lay hands on the sick, and they shall recover" (Mark 16:17–18). And from John 14:12: "He that believeth on me, the works that I do shall he do also; and greater works than these shall he do; because I go unto my Father."

Watch Out for "Sappers"

Yogis have known for centuries that being in the presence of negative persons is a draining experience and should be avoided if one's vital energy or life force is to be preserved. Now this theory is being echoed by neuropsychiatrist Shafica Karagulla in her book *Breakthrough to Creativity: Your Higher Sense Perception.*

Dr. Karagulla is a member of the Royal College of Physicians of Edinburgh, the highest medical qualification in Britain, and came to the United States to do research in abnormal mental states. *Breakthrough to Creativity* is a fascinating account of a scientifically oriented psychiatrist's research into what most of us call extrasensory perception.

Dr. Karagulla tells of "sensitives" who can see the energy field surrounding the body and describes what happens to this field of energy when people encounter negative individuals whom she calls sappers. The sapper is a self-centered individual, enclosed in his own orbit, who lacks outgoingness to other people and the outside world. These people do not generate their own energy but are psychological parasites, using the physical, mental, and emotional energies of other people. A sensitive can actually see the sapper draining the life force from his victim.

In the presence of a sapper the victim feels increasingly tired and irritable and has an overwhelming urge to get away from the sapper. Unfortunately, the sapper is often a member of one's family, so getting away produces a feeling of guilt, and the victim returns for yet another energy drain. Some sappers can pull energy from anyone, whereas others drain only specific victims.

If encounters with certain people consistently leave you drained, irritable, and resentful, there is a good chance that that person is a sapper who is tapping your vital energy. Mothers of young children know this drained feeling all too well, because youngsters are sappers until they are old enough to be aware of the feelings of others; fortunately, most of them outgrow this form of immaturity.

If your life is plagued by a sapper, and if you can't completely avoid the person, at least protect yourself from this psychic sponge. Visualize yourself surrounded by a large plastic dome that is impervious to the attack of negative parasites, and mentally affirm that your vital energy and positive attitudes will remain intact. Positive mental energy is one of the greatest gifts of life—don't squander it!

3

BREATH IS LIFE

Of all aspects of yoga, the breathing techniques are the most difficult to master without the guidance of a trained teacher. Without these breathing techniques, however, yoga would be just another method of physical fitness. It is this special breathing, called pranayama, that enables yoga practitioners to control not only the body, but more importantly, the mind.

Breathing is an automatic process, one that we normally do without thinking about it, and only when we are troubled with asthma, emphysema, allergies, or a cold are we completely aware of how vital the breathing process really is. The human body can go without food for unlimited periods of time, and without water for a lesser time, but without air, life terminates in a few short minutes.

In yoga, breathing is considered so paramount that the yogi measures life not in the number of years lived, but in the number of breaths allotted for each incarnation, or lifetime. If a person breathes hurriedly, the allocation of breaths is used up sooner, and life ends prematurely. Though long life is generally a universal goal, it is often insufficient motivation to induce people to learn breath control *right now*. Swami Rama, an Indian yogi with ashrams and training centers throughout the United States, relates experiences that explain why controlled breathing is of such importance in India.

Trained to be a yogi from age three, Swami Rama can breathe in such a way that there is no apparent evidence of the breathing process. There is no movement of chest or abdomen, and the breathing cannot be detected at the nostrils. In the bear-infested region of the Himalayas where he grew up, this form of breathing was a must for survival. Upon encountering a bear, the budding swami learned to lie down, suspend normal breathing, and remain motionless. The bears sniff the nostrils and mouth and attack if there is evidence of life. When no breath is detected, the bears assume the person is dead and do not attack.

What Yoga Breathing Will Do for You

No such motivation exists in the United States, where encounters with bears are, to say the least, infrequent. Here, the most beneficial effects of breath control are relief from tension, prevention of disease, control of such negative emotions as anger, impatience, and nervousness, and learning the art of concentration. Your state of mind is reflected in your breathing. When you're angry, nervous, and upset, your breathing is rapid and shallow. Normal breathing returns only when you calm down. And anyone can discern whether or not a person is asleep by observing that person's breathing. Only during sleep does the average person breathe properly, an indication of the relationship between breathing and relaxation.

Mastery of yoga breathing will allow you to control your emotions rather than being controlled by them. Instead of waiting for the emotions, and then the breathing, to return to normal, by consciously controlling the breathing, you will also bring the emotions under your conscious control.

Yoga breathing is the exact opposite of the manner in which most people breathe, and I would like to emphasize the word *most*. When I first read about yoga breathing methods, I found them confusing, because the literature stated that it was the opposite of the way people normally breathed. I have always breathed in the yoga manner, and there are others who have also done so.

The Nose Is for Breathing, the Mouth Is for Eating

Of all the animals, only man—with his logical mind and perverted instincts —is a mouth breather. And he is not intended to be. When man breathes through his mouth, he thwarts the built-in security system that was intended to guard his most precious possession—the respiratory system. Simple as it looks, the nose is a complex mechanism. When we breathe properly, air enters through the two nostrils, these nostrils being separated by a thin wall of cartilage and bones called the septum.

Just inside the nostrils grow short coarse hairs, the outer security guards that filter out large dust particles and an occasional insect. Farther back are two tunnels, the nasal passages, lined with mucous membranes covered with microscopic, hairlike projections called cilia. The constantly moving cilia, which are destroyed by smoking, move dust-laden mucus into the throat so that it bypasses the lungs. This mucus also kills some germs and stops the growth of others.

Each nasal passage also contains three turbinates that warm incoming air, and between the turbinates are humidity-control centers to assure proper moisture in the air headed for the lungs. Mouth breathers forgo the benefits of this marvelous security system and leave themselves wide open for a host of respiratory problems.

Once in the lungs, which are composed of millions of tiny air cells, inhaled oxygen comes into contact with the blood. The lungs cleanse and purify the blood that carries the waste products of the human system. We breathe in oxygen, it unites with the blood, and the blood releases waste products that we breathe out in the form of carbon dioxide. This is an impressive cooperative system and so automatic that we fail to appreciate it fully.

The blood, purified by its intake of oxygen and the releasing of carbon dioxide, returns by way of the arteries to nourish all the cells of the body and brain. Each cell is first nourished by the oxygen-laden blood, then relinquishes its burden of waste products that is transported back to the lungs via the veins. Outgoing purified arterial blood is bright red, fresh, and full of life-giving qualities. On the return trip, venous blood reflects the load of impurities it carries in its dark, bluish color.

You may never have given your cells a second thought, and that's probably a good thing if you're overwhelmed by numbers. The cell is the basic unit of life, and you have more than a million million of them. Cells are specialists. Some form liver tissue, others make up muscle tissue, and still others form nerve tissue. Each cell is alive—as alive as you are. Like you, each cell "breathes," takes in food, and gets rid of wastes. And, like all living things, cells die. In fact, every minute about three billion cells in your body die and are immediately replaced by three billion new cells born by a special division process called mitosis. The health of every one of these cells is affected by the way you breathe.

The lungs are large, pyramid-shaped organs made up of masses of spongy tissue. The entire lung was designed to be used in the vital breathing process; unfortunately, most people use only about one-third of it. Take a deep breathe, and see what happens. Most people inhale by thrusting out the chest and pulling in the abdomen. This is incorrect. Learning how to breathe properly is the first step on the path to self-realization through yoga.

The lungs rest on the diaphragm, the dome-shaped muscle that separates the chest cavity from the abdominal area. In order to completely fill the lungs, the diaphragm must be lowered to provide necessary space for lung expansion. Thrusting out the chest while inhaling leaves the diaphragm uninvolved, utilizes only the upper third of the lung structure, and is called high breathing. Pulling in the abdomen pushes the diaphragm still higher and compresses the lungs. Persons breathing in this manner must take more breaths, because they do not obtain enough oxygen in each breath.

Another form of incomplete breathing is called middle breathing, in which the rib cage expands sideways during inhalation. This utilizes, perhaps, the upper two-thirds of the lung and is more efficient than high breathing but is still less than ideal.

In low breathing, also called abdominal, deep, or diaphragmatic breathing, the abdomen pushes out with each inhalation, lowering the diaphragm and allowing the lower lung to fill with oxygen. This is better than high and middle breathing because it activates the lower and generally unused portion of the lung.

Best of all is complete yoga breathing, which activates the entire lung structure. To learn complete yoga breathing, we must learn low, middle, and high breathing, and then put them all together. To learn low breathing, lie down on the floor or a mat, relax, and place both hands on the abdomen with the tips of the index and longest fingers of one hand against the tips of the corresponding fingers on the other hand. Inhale, and push the abdomen out as you inhale. If you are doing this properly, the tips of the fingers will pull apart as you inhale and come back together as you exhale.

This low, or diaphragmatic, breathing should be done only three or four times during each practice session, then resume breathing in your normal fashion. Low breathing pulls a much greater supply of oxygen into the system, and when the system is unaccustomed to such an increased amount, a condition known as hyperventilation will result if breathing deeply is carried to extremes. Hyperventilation produces an unpleasant sensation of dizziness and perhaps even nausea. Repeat the three or four abdominal breaths several times during the day for at least a week or two so that you become adept at this manner of breathing and so that your system becomes accustomed to the greater oxygen supply.

Although complete yoga breathing utilizes high, middle, and low breathing, these methods must be learned in steps to make sure each step is correct before proceeding to the next. Middle breathing, also called intercostal breathing, is a form of breathing taught to emphysema patients by inhalation therapists. To activate the middle section of the lung, sit, kneel, or stand, and place the hands on the lower side of the rib cage, fingers somewhat spread apart on the front side of the body, thumbs pointing toward each other in back. Concentrate on the middle section of the lungs where the hands are placed. Inhale, and expand the rib cage sideward as you do, resisting slightly with the hands. Exhale, and push the rib cage back in again. The grip with the hands should be quite firm, and the movement of breathing should be easily felt in the hands. Practice this form of breathing from one to two weeks before going on to the complete breathing. High breathing is the way you probably breathe normally. It occurs when the chest expands upon inhalation and the rest of the lungs remain inactive.

Complete Yoga Breathing

Having learned the elements of breathing in steps, we will now try to put them together in one continuous flowing movement. Sit or stand, and relax the abdomen, allowing it to push out as you begin inhaling. Continue breathing in, and be aware of the sides of the rib cage expanding. Keep inhaling until there is no more available space in the lungs to fill. Try to avoid lifting the shoulders at the end of this process. To exhale, visualize your lungs as a glass of water that can only be emptied from top to bottom. Begin exhaling through the nose, emptying the top of the lungs, then the middle, and finally pull the abdomen in to push the last bit of stale air from the bottom of the lungs.

Although slow, deep inhalation is important, exhalation is considered even more so because this process rids the lungs of accumulated impurities. Those who exhale shallowly have lungs that are inactive, the lower section never quite ridding itself of old stagnant air. Unless the old air is completely exhaled, there is insufficient room for fresh air. Without sufficient oxygen all of the body's cells lack vitality.

Many breathing exercises are described in detail later in this chapter, but complete yoga breathing must be mastered before going to the specific exercises. Complete yoga breathing requires concentrated effort when you first begin; eventually, in a month, two months, or a year, you will suddenly realize that you are automatically breathing this way all the time.

The Meaning of Hatha

Yoga breathing is such an integral part of the system that the name *hatha* refers to this breathing process. *Ha* means sun, referring to the breath that enters the right nostril that heats the body; *tha* means moon, and the left nostril inhales the cooling moon breath.

Earlier in this chapter, I discussed the physiological aspects of our breathing process, the nourishing of cells through inhalation and the elimination of waste products through exhalation. These facts apply to the physical body, are common knowledge throughout the world, and represent the exoteric explanation of the respiratory process. They can be understood by the general public and are not restricted to an inner circle of scholars or disciples.

The Principle and Meaning of Prana

Hatha-yoga, however, presents an esoteric theory regarding respiration, a theory reserved for a select few disciples, which was closely guarded for centuries and handed down from guru to student only after years of discipline. This theory is the principle of *prana*. Just as oxygen is used by the physical body, prana is the universal energy force for the astral body.

The astral body is an exact duplicate of the physical, except that it is of a subtler substance and is not subject to the same limitations as the physical body. Some schools of thought maintain that dreams, particularly when the dreams are in color, are actually experiences of the astral body. Just as dogs can hear some sounds that are of too high a frequency to be detected by human ears, the astral body vibrations are invisible to all but highly clairvoyant individuals. The astral body, which is of a higher dimension, is said to be connected to the physical body by a thin cord that remains intact throughout life. Highly advanced occultists claim to be able to project their astral body to any point on earth, or beyond, at will.

The known senses of sight, hearing, touch, taste, and smell are senses of the physical body, whereas extrasensory perception and so-called supernormal powers are the province of the astral body. The physical body is nourished by food, water, and oxygen, and the astral body survives through prana. Both bodies coexist, and although they are for different purposes, both are controlled by the mind.

The subtlety of prana eludes even our most sophisticated measuring and analyzing devices. It is in air, in water, in food, and in all of the cells of our body, and yet it is not of the same chemical makeup as any of them. Although prana exists in all things, it is most readily available in the air we breathe. It is useful even to those who have never heard of prana.

The child stumbles and falls, skinning a knee in the process. The knife slips and cuts the finger of the harried housewife. And the weekend carpenter takes faulty aim and suffers a smashed thumb. All three react instinctively, and similarly.

The child takes a deep breath and cups the injured knee between both hands. The housewife takes a deep breath and pushes the cut together in an apparent effort to stem the bleeding. And the hammer's victim, usually

after uttering a profanity or two, takes a deep breath and clasps the throb-
bing digit with the other hand.

These reactions are automatic and intuitive, and yet they underscore a
basic concept of yoga—the theory of prana. Prana is the Sanskrit word
for absolute energy, and it is the energy of the universe, the life force in all
elements of our world, and it is all around us. Placing the hands around
an injury is a subconscious effort to transfer this energy that permeates
the body to the spot that hurts.

Intuition, in yoga, is thought to be the memory of the soul. Those acts
that we do intuitively, such as the deep breath that immediately follows a
safety-threatening incident, seem to indicate an understanding of the cosmic laws governing our universe. When more life force is needed, the subconscious prods each of us to take a deep breath, increasing the prana in
the system. The public speaker, in the throes of stage fright, instinctively
takes a deep breath as he approaches the podium, absorbing more prana
to calm the nervous system.

An adequate supply of oxygen and prana in the system is so vital that
it is not left to chance. The child whose temper tantrum leads to holding
the breath will faint and resume normal breathing before oxygen starva-
tion causes brain damage.

An adequate supply of prana in the system is just as important as oxygen. It is reflected in a sound nervous system and an aura of vitality, mag-
netism, or charisma. Many of the world's charmers possess, unknowingly,
great command of prana, and they seem to others to be full of life, have
great strength of personality, and magnetize all who come within their
orbit.

Prana is stored throughout the body, but the primary storage center is
the solar plexus. When a mother comforts a child by holding that child to
her body, she is intuitively trying to transfer prana—her life force—to her
offspring. Cradling an injured or frightened pet against you is another such
effort. And faith healers or Christian Science healers utilize prana in their
healing efforts. The laying on of hands, suspect as it is in some circles, is
merely a transfer of prana from a strong person to a weaker one. We all
do this to a greater or lesser degree when we try to comfort or reassure
others by touching them. Like the biblical reference to bread cast upon
the waters, the more you give away, the more you have—particularly if
you are aware of absorbing prana with every breath you take.

The earlier brief description of the physical process of breathing recalled
the respiratory system, which includes the nostrils and nasal passages that
transport oxygen to the lungs. From the lungs, oxygen is supplied to all
parts of the body through the bloodstream via arteries and capillaries. A
network of veins returns the blood to the lungs. This explains how oxygen
nourishes the physical body and disposes of its waste products.

Prana enters the system through the same passages and is distributed to all parts of the body through luminous canals called *nadis*, which are to the astral body what veins and arteries are to the physical body. The astral body contains numerous nadis, but the three main ones are named *ida*, *pingala*, and *sushumna*.

The most important nadi, the sushumna, is said to be located in the center of the spinal canal, and the ida (pronounced eeda) and pingala intersect it like the intertwining snakes of Mercury's caduceus. The kundalini power (the serpent power that lies coiled at the base of the spine), discussed in the next chapter, which is located in the lowermost muladhara chakra, is released when the nadis are purified, and this serpent power travels through the sushumna nadi activating the various chakras. It is interesting to note that the caduceus is the symbol of the medical profession, the intertwining snakes representing wisdom. In yoga the releasing of the kundalini power, the serpent power, is credited with expanded states of consciousness, extrasensory perception, telepathy, and clairvoyance. Keep in mind that all of this is connected with the breathing process.

Breath through the right nostril, the *ha* or heating sun breath, is connected to the pingala nadi, and the ida nadi relates to the left nostril breath, the *tha* or cooling moon breath. At any given time, the inhaled breath flows through one of the nostrils more freely than the other. You can check this yourself by closing the left nostril and breathing through the right; then reversing it, closing the right nostril and breathing through the left. You will notice that the inhalation process is much easier through one nostril.

In the normal, healthy person this ease of inhalation changes from one nostril to the other approximately every two hours—more precisely, every hour and fifty minutes. When the breathing remains primarily through one nostril for more than two hours, it indicates an abnormality in some part of the body. When this breath remains unchanged for twenty-four hours, yogis claim it heralds an impending illness, the seriousness of which is related to the length of time the breath centers in one nostril. The alternate breathing exercise outlined later in this chapter is a specific for controlling proper breath through the nostrils.

In our fast-paced society one of the greatest benefits of yoga breathing is its effectiveness in relieving tension. It is a tranquilizer, but a natural one, and has no bad side effects. You can use it anytime, anywhere, and it's free. Concentration is enhanced when tension is eliminated, and yoga breathing can also be used as a quick pickup when you're tired.

Breathing Exercises in Your Daily Program

Yoga breathing can be done at any time, but it should be included at the end of your daily asana (exercise) program, just before the complete relaxation. After each asana, lie down and do the complete yoga breathing until the muscles and the breathing rate are back to normal. Then before the complete relaxation, do some of the specific breathing exercises such as rhythmic breathing, alternate breathing, and cosmic breathing. Incidentally, breathing exercises that include holding the breath, and the more strenuous asanas, should be avoided by anyone taking antibiotics.

RHYTHMIC BREATHING—EXERCISE #1

According to the Bible, the book of Ecclesiastes, "To every thing there is a season, and a time to every purpose under the heaven. A time to be born, and a time to die. . . . A time to weep, and a time to laugh; a time to mourn, and a time to dance. . . . A time to keep silence, and a time to speak." These lines reflect the basic underlying rhythm that affects everything in the universe.

Each of the planets has its own rhythm, this word from the Greek *rhythmos*, meaning measured motion. Night follows day in precise order, the seasons march in orderly procession, and even each cell of our bodies is destiny-linked to the cosmic timetable. Consider the infinite planning that provides a 13-day life-span for a white blood cell and 120 days for a red one, liver cells that are allotted eighteen months, and nerve cells that can live one hundred years.

Just as each body cell is timed to harmonize with the whole organism, so this whole organism is linked, in a unique fashion, to the universe. Yogis maintain that the rhythmic breathing that follows is the method of attuning individual man to his outer environment, to the universe.

Rhythmic breathing calms the mind and body, particularly the nervous system. It familiarizes each person with his or her own internal timer, and rhythmic breathing has more power than erratic breathing. Compare this form of breathing with the rhythmic marching of soldiers. Marchers must break step and rhythm when crossing a bridge, or the powerful en masse steps would create such vibrations that the bridge could not withstand them. Regular steps, lacking the power of rhythm and vibration, leave the bridge unharmed. Breathe rhythmically for increased inner power.

To breathe rhythmically, sit or lie down with spine straight, and place the fingertips on the wrist to determine your heartbeat. When this rhythm is familiar to you, inhale a comfortable breath while counting the pulse beats. Let's assume the count is four, an average number. To breathe rhythmically, inhale while counting four pulse beats, then exhale while counting four pulse beats. This is a round; start by performing six rounds. As your lung capacity increases, add another pulse beat so you will be inhaling for five beats and exhaling for five beats. Increase count gradually.

RHYTHMIC BREATHING WITH RETENTION—EXERCISE #2

After doing the rhythmic breathing for a while, you will be so familiar with your own inner rhythm that it will be unnecessary to keep the fingers on the pulse. When this form of breathing has become comfortable for you, and after you have increased your initial count by at least a heartbeat or two, it is time to add another step in the breathing process called retention. Retention is the holding of the breath for specified lengths of time after inhalation and pausing for that same length of time after the exhalation in each round. In other words, you will inhale, retain, exhale, retain, during each round. The retention, or holding, time is always half the inhaling and exhaling time in this breathing exercise.

Let's assume that your rhythmic breathing count has increased to six. Utilizing the retention, you will inhale for six pulse beats, hold for three pulse beats, exhale for six beats, and hold the lungs empty for three beats. Start with six rounds of rhythmic breathing with retention, and work up *gradually* as your capacity increases. In working toward increased capacity, first start increasing the number of rounds you perform. This can be as few as ten rounds or as many as sixty.

As you become more proficient in the breathing, you will eventually experience the feeling that six counts is not long enough to take as deep a breath as you would like. When this happens, it is time to add to your number of counts. Accordingly, you will then go to eight pulse beats for inhalation and exhalation, and half that, four beats, for the retention period. As in the initial rhythmic breathing, first increase the number of rounds you perform, and eventually add additional beats maintaining the 2 to 1 ratio between inhalation and exhalation and the retention period.

SINGLE NOSTRIL BREATHING WITHOUT RETENTION— EXERCISE #3

Much of yoga must be experienced to be believed, and a gradual introduction to the rhythmic breathing is usually sufficient to demonstrate to the beginner the effect of breathing on the nervous system. Once that has been mastered, you are ready to learn alternate breathing, which begins with single nostril breathing and which will emphasize the exhalation process. Keep in mind that unless the lungs are fully emptied of old air, there is insufficient room in the lungs to take a complete breath of fresh air.

The human adult lung capacity is about three to four quarts of air, a normal inhalation taking in about a pint, a normal exhalation releasing an equal amount. Even after death, the average lungs contain more than a quart of air. Fear or similar emotions increase the need for oxygen, and a breath taken then may measure two and a half quarts instead of the usual pint, a meager amount considering the job it has to do.

In single nostril breathing, remember that the air normally flows more freely through one or the other nostril, this free flow changing approximately every two hours. This may cause you to feel that you are not getting enough air when using one nostril. In single nostril breathing, in which the exhalation count is twice the inhalation count, it is important that you pace your exhalation so that you will have enough air to last throughout the count. To do this, it sometimes helps to imagine that you are exhaling through a straw.

Sit on the floor or a mat with spine straight and legs crossed tailor fashion. Later, when you have learned them, you will want to use one of the meditative postures, such as the Lotus or Half Lotus, for breathing exercises. Maintain an erect posture with shoulders back and chin parallel to the floor. Close the right nostril with the right thumb, and inhale to a count of four through the left nostril. Then, without retention, exhale to a count of eight through the same nostril. This is one round. Start by performing ten rounds with the right nostril closed.

After the tenth round, close the left nostril with the ring finger and little finger of the right hand, and repeat ten rounds inhaling and exhaling through the right nostril. Practice this breathing exercise for one week or more, until it is comfortable for you, before going on to the next breathing exercise.

ALTERNATE BREATHING WITHOUT RETENTION— EXERCISE #4

The single nostril breathing is a preliminary for the alternate breathing in which air is inhaled through one nostril and exhaled through the other. Once you have progressed to this alternate breathing, the single nostril breathing is unnecessary, since it is just one step in the more advanced alternate breathing. It is, however, a necessary preliminary and one that must be done easily before proceeding.

Sit in an erect posture as before, and close the right nostril with the right thumb. Inhale to a count of four through the left nostril, then without pausing, close the left nostril with ring finger and little finger, and exhale to a count of eight through the right nostril. This is half a round. Without pausing, inhale to a count of four through the right nostril, then close the right nostril with the thumb, and exhale through the left nostril to a count of eight. This completes the round.

Although this form of breathing is measured in rounds, and you can keep track of the rounds by counting on your left hand, there is no pause between the rounds. To the casual observer it would appear to be one continuous process. Start with ten rounds; as you become more proficient in alternate breathing, increase the number of rounds to twenty or so. Then, as in the previous exercises, begin increasing the count for each inhalation and exhalation, inhaling to a count of five and exhaling to a count of ten, inhaling for six counts and exhaling for twelve, etc. Inhalation is always half the exhalation count, the ratio of 1 to 2 being maintained.

COMPLETE ALTERNATE BREATHING
WITH RETENTION—EXERCISE #5

Complete alternate breathing, with retention, is one of the most powerful and effective of all yoga breathing exercises. It is a basic breathing exercise and replaces the two previous exercises, which are merely preliminaries for this all-important one. *Persons suffering from high blood pressure or heart disorders should not hold the breath.* They may do Exercise #4, which is without retention. Contact lenses should be removed when performing breathing exercises with retention to avoid bloodshot eyes.

This exercise has both an exoteric and an esoteric value. The physiological effect is easily recognized, because this exercise is probably nature's greatest tranquilizer. Use it whenever you are upset or nervous as well as in your daily practice. Its calming effect is immediately felt in the physical body and nervous system.

On the esoteric level, where the astral body is involved, alternate breathing is unsurpassed for purifying the nadis, the tubular channels through which prana is distributed throughout the astral body. This purification of the nadis is necessary before going on to more advanced pranayama. Without prior purification, some exercises do not produce the intended effects. The purification process requires varying lengths of time for different people, but body perspiration is the first stage of purification. As the nadis become more purified, a tremor will be felt in the body; this is a normal reaction and is not cause for alarm.

Sit in Lotus, Half Lotus, or cross-legged posture, making sure that the spine is kept straight with the shoulders back. (These positions are shown in the photo section of Chapter 4.) The left hand rests on the left knee, the left thumb and forefinger forming a circle with the thumb on top. The palm is up between sunrise and sunset, down between sunset and sunrise. Close the right nostril with the right thumb (as shown on page 41), and inhale to a count of four through the left nostril. Keeping the thumb in place, completely close the nostrils by placing the right ring finger and little finger against the left nostril, and hold for a count of sixteen. Now remove the thumb only, and exhale to a count of eight through the right nostril. Inhale through the right nostril to a count of four; close both nostrils for a count of sixteen; remove ring and little fingers, and exhale to a count of eight through the left nostril. This is one round. The correct ratio of inhalation, retention, and exhalation is 1:4:2. However, if the retention period is too difficult, you may begin by using a ratio of 1:2:2. In other words, inhale for a count of four, retain for a count of eight, and exhale for a count of eight. Start with ten rounds, and work up to twenty rounds gradually.

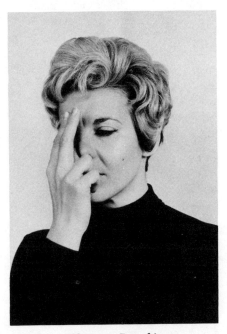

Alternate Breathing

In all of the breathing exercises it is important to remember that each person is unique, and breathing capacity differs among people. If the instructions for these exercises seem difficult, perform fewer rounds, and do not continue if you become tired. You will find that your capacity will increase as you perform the exercises each day.

After you can do twenty rounds of alternate breathing easily, begin adding to the number of counts used. For example, after 4:16:8 is accomplished without difficulty or strain, increase the count to 5:20:10. Here you will inhale to a count of five, retain the breath for twenty counts, and exhale to a count of ten. Increase the count gradually, and do not go beyond 8:32:16. The breath should never be retained for more than thirty-two counts by any but the most highly advanced students.

COSMIC BREATHING—EXERCISE #6

Cosmic breathing is not one of the classic breathing exercises, but it is a favorite with all the classes I have taught. I am indebted to my good friend, Adelinde Ostermann, an excellent teacher and director of the Toronto (Canada) Yoga Center, for sharing it with me. This exercise teams up the complete yoga breath with various arm movements. It accentuates positive thinking by linking constructive thoughts to the breathing process. Yoga is concerned with physical, mental, and spiritual development, and a round of cosmic breathing is devoted to each.

The power of the mind is vast and fascinating, particularly when it operates with the concentration provided by yoga breathing. It is yours to use for the establishment of the kind of life you want. Long the theme of positive thinkers, this concept has been ridiculed by the skeptics. But the importance of controlling the way you think is gradually gaining acceptance. The medical profession has now linked various personality traits to those individuals they have designated as prone to cancer, heart disease, and ulcers. This cosmic breathing exercise can help change your attitudes and your general health. Follow the illustration below and directions on opposite page.

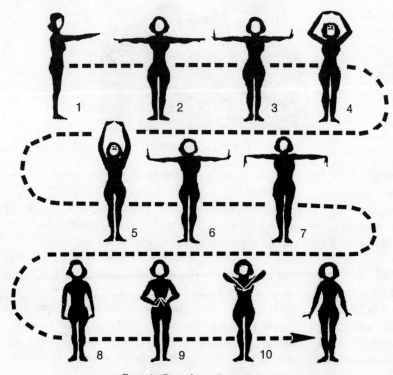

Cosmic Breathing Exercises

1. Stand erect with legs together and arms held relaxed at sides. Inhale, and at the same time raise both arms straight out in front of you until they are parallel to the floor at shoulder height, elbows straight, fingers straight and together, palms pointing to the floor. Inhale thoughts of a sound physical body.

2. Exhale, bringing the arms sideward at right angles to the body, still at shoulder level, palms down. Exhale all ill health.

3. In one *sharp* motion bend the hands at the wrists until fingers point toward the ceiling. The hands are now at right angles to the arms.

4. Inhale, slowly raise the eyes toward the ceiling, and at the same time bring the hands upward in a semicircular motion until the middle fingers touch about four to six inches above the eyes, palms up. Inhale tranquillity.

5. Exhale, pushing the palms toward the ceiling. Make this an extreme stretching motion, stretching both the arms and the spine. The eyes are still focused on the backs of the hands at this point. Exhale tension.

6. Inhale, slowly bringing the face back to original position and bringing the arms back to the same position they were in after completing Step 3. Arms are parallel to the floor, fingers pointing toward the ceiling. Inhale temperance.

7. In one *sharp* movement bend the hands at the wrists until fingers are pointing toward the floor.

8. Exhale while bringing the straightened arms downward toward the floor. Exhale intemperance.

9. When the extended fingers are about a foot apart, begin inhaling as the arms continue toward each other. Continue inhaling, and begin pointing fingers toward the ceiling so that you can place the hands together, back to back, fingers pointed to ceiling. Raise the hands together in this position until they are just under the chin. Inhale thoughts of sound nutrition.

10. Exhale as you reverse the hands so fingers point toward the floor, and bring the hands down toward the floor still back to back. The hands will part naturally at a certain point, and the arms should be brought back to the sides of the body, hands bent at the wrists, palms facing the floor. Exhale unnatural food cravings.

Repeat the entire exercise three times.

During the second round, which stresses good mental attitudes:
Inhale positive thoughts; exhale negativity.
Inhale an even temper; exhale irritability.
Inhale maturity; exhale immaturity.
Inhale generosity; exhale envy.

During the third round, for spiritual growth, concentrate on:
Inhaling love; exhaling hatred.
Inhaling contentment; exhaling greed.
Inhaling wisdom; exhaling prejudice.
Inhaling truth; exhaling dishonesty.

YOGI CLEANSING BREATH—EXERCISE #7

This exercise also emphasizes the exhalation process. When the lungs are cleansed of their accumulated impurities through this breath, an instant "pickup," or recharge, is felt as each cell of the body receives a fresh supply of invigorating oxygen. Here are the directions:

1. Stand or sit in cross-legged or meditative posture, keeping the spine straight. Inhale a complete yoga breath through the nose, and retain it for a few seconds.

2. Pucker up the lips as if you were going to whistle, then vigorously exhale a short burst of air through the pursed lips; pause for a second or two, and exhale another short burst of air. Continue in this fashion, exhaling, pausing, exhaling, and pausing until the lungs are completely empty.

3. Perform ten to twenty rounds, increasing the number of rounds gradually.

INVIGORATING BREATH—EXERCISE #8

This exercise stresses low, middle, and high breathing in sequence and couples breath intake with vigorous arm movements. It also eases tension from the back and shoulder-blade area and loosens lower back and hamstrings. Directions:

1. Stand erect, being aware of the posture. The spine is straight, buttocks tucked in, shoulders back, and arms hang straight at the sides. You will be inhaling through the nostrils in three short inhalations and exhaling once through the mouth.

2. Inhale a deep abdominal breath, and at the same time, sharply extend the straightened arms out in front of you until arms are at shoulder height, palms pointing toward the floor.

3. Inhale again, filling the middle section of the lungs and briskly extending the arms sideways as far as they will go, again at shoulder level.

4. Inhale once more, this time moving the arms vigorously over the head until the palms touch and the arms remain straight. This inhalation fills the upper section of the lungs.

5. Then completely relax the body, exhale through the mouth as you let the upper body fall forward like a limp rag doll. The bending should come from the lowest part of the spine below the waist, and your arms and neck

should be relaxed and the hands will touch, or nearly touch, the floor.
Repeat several times.

How to Use the Breathing with the Asanas

In the following chapter on asanas, the inhalation and exhalation is
indicated for each exercise, and this should be the complete yoga breath,
Exercise #1. Although pranayama is the fourth step in hatha-yoga, after
the asanas, the breathing should be incorporated with the exercises for
maximum benefits.

4

THE ASANAS—
HOW TO GET STARTED

Yoga places people in three categories—sleeping, awakened, or enlightened. The fact that you are reading this book is an indication that you are in the awakened group.

The sleeping individual may be successful, happy, and satisfied with life, but he accepts only what can be seen, touched, tasted, and proved. In other words, he uses only his five senses and is unaware of anything beyond this. The awakened person knows he has tapped only a minute portion of his potential. This person knows the universe contains more than the five senses, and he tries to develop beyond these. Persons involved in yoga are awakened and are trying to learn to control the body and, ultimately, the mind. To be enlightened is yoga's goal. Enlightened man has reached his potential, controls the latent forces within him, and uses them to his advantage.

How to Learn Yoga

In learning the art and science of yoga you can either join a class or teach yourself at home. Should you elect to join a class, it is vitally important that you select your teacher with care. Even though teachers may teach exactly the same asanas in a lesson, any class will reflect its teacher's approach to yoga. Yoga is a system of physical, mental, and spiritual development, and most teachers consciously or unconsciously stress one of these elements more than the other two.

One teacher may place the highest emphasis on physical development, dwelling mostly on the physical benefits to be gained from each posture and touching lightly, if at all, on mental and spiritual development. Another teacher may ask the class to assume a posture and then urge the participants to concentrate the mind in specific ways. Still others may underplay the physical or mental benefits and lead the students toward more spiritual or mystical experiences. The best teachers strive for balance in these three areas.

Some yoga classes have almost a religious solemnity, some are primarily practical, and others have an atmosphere of humor and joy. Each type can be good, depending on what the individual is seeking.

The Importance of Teacher Certification

The upsurge of interest in yoga in recent years has resulted in classes being taught by many persons who have not been trained to teach. Should you enroll in a class offered by a YMCA or YWCA or similar organization, inquire about the qualifications of the yoga teacher.

Indra Devi–trained teachers receive certificates based on the results of written and oral exams as well as many hours of teaching experience under the supervision of Indra Devi herself. If a teacher does not have a certificate from her or another master yoga teacher, it should be ascertained where he or she was trained and for how long.

Swami Rama also is an excellent trainer of teachers. Many of the larger cities have teacher-training centers that he has established, and the teachers he trains reflect his own high standards of excellence.

There are undoubtedly many other fine teacher-training centers, but I mention only these two because I have been through their classes and have firsthand experience with them.

A yoga program can be tailored for almost anyone, regardless of age and physical condition, but an untrained teacher or one inadequately trained may not be aware of the physical hazards of some postures for people with specific illnesses or chronic conditions.

One of the saddest consequences of unskilled teaching is that many students are turned off, thinking that the bungled and erroneous viewpoint they received is all there is to yoga—and beginners have no criteria with which to judge their classes. One so-called teacher, intrigued solely by the profit motive, admitted that she didn't care if her students ever came back to class—after they had paid her.

Beware also of the gym-teacher approach. Yoga is a gentle, passive approach to physical fitness, and if a class resembles a gymnastics class, it may be exercise, but it isn't yoga.

Responsibility of Teacher to Student

When Indra Devi teaches a yoga class, one feels she has just discovered a fantastic body of knowledge that she gives to you as one might present a precious jewel.

Far from being a recent convert to yoga, at seventy-four she has been teaching yoga and training teachers for more than thirty years. She remains fresh, enthusiastic, spontaneous, and untiring. Mataji lives up to her own high standards for teachers—yoga is an integral part of her life, and she spreads the word with a missionary zeal.

In emphasizing yoga's noncompetitiveness, she compares a class to a bouquet of flowers, stressing each person's uniqueness. "While you may be a perfect daisy, you will never be a rose and must always be yourself, developing your own best abilities," she advises.

"A good yoga teacher must love people, but no one can love everybody. You cannot give what you do not have, but you can at least give attention, time, and patience to all your students. Before and after class you may be friends with your students; during class you are teacher and student."

A good teacher knows the subject and, more important, knows how to teach it. Beautiful performance of the asanas is useless unless you are capable of instructing others to do them. The teacher should demonstrate the asana, or have an assistant demonstrate it, then check to make sure that each student is performing it correctly.

The teacher should be careful to present facts accurately and must set a good example in manners, behavior, and dress. The size of a class depends upon the teacher, but each student should receive individual attention. Mataji also warns that yoga classes often regard their teacher as a combination doctor, priest, and psychiatrist—which is a heady experience and also a tremendous responsibility.

Being a firm believer in the power of the Universal Mind, Divine Intelligence, or God—call it what you wish—I mentally repeat an affirmation before each class that I will be aware of the needs of my students, spoken or unspoken, and that Divine Intelligence will provide the correct answers to any and all questions. Some of my answers to questions surprise even me.

One example of this occurred when a young woman asked why the front of her neck hurt when she did the Shoulder Stand. I explained that normal everyday activities seldom called for the chin to be pressed firmly into the base of the neck, and she was feeling an unaccustomed pressure in that area, and then I added, "Unless you're a Taurus, and if you are a Taurus, you should have your doctor check it at once." This young Taurus had an undetected tumor on the thyroid and fortunately heeded my advice, possibly saving her life.

A yoga class generally contains a good cross section of people and personalities, positive thinkers as well as those emotionally crippled by negative self-images. The feelings of incompetence engendered by destructive early programming lead to lives of unrealized potential, and a yoga class should guarantee success, if only in one small segment of life. Although a yoga class isn't going to completely upgrade anyone's self-esteem, it can provide some assistance in the building of confidence. It's a shock to see people who feel they have never succeeded at anything. Therefore, a sensitive and experienced teacher will make certain that each person in the class succeeds to the limit of his or her physical ability.

Everybody Finds His Own Thing

It is axiomatic that in any series of classes every person will find some posture that he or she does better than anyone else in the class. By observing areas of strength and flexibility, a good teacher can lead students to such successes without creating a competitive situation.

Beginning students must look beyond the physical flexibility of their teacher for an even greater attribute—a flexible mind. Those who have been certified and have been teaching for several years must be on guard against developing the feeling that they know everything there is to know about yoga. When your field is human potential, how can learning ever stop?

Your Teacher Is Programming You

The final ten or fifteen minutes of a yoga class are devoted to complete relaxation. Contrary to common belief, relaxation is not an automatic result of passivity but is an active process in which the mind urges each part of the body in turn to relax. The eyes are closed, the eyelids relaxed, and the instructor gently and slowly urges: "Relax your toes. . . . Relax your calves. . . . Concentrate on the backs of your thighs, and tell them to relax." This controlled relaxation continues through all the parts of the body, the internal organs, and finally the mind. The tension that permeates the fiber of our society oozes away, producing a relaxed sense of euphoria and well-being.

The mind must remain blank; when thoughts come, they should be brushed gently but firmly away. The mind is compared to a calm pool of water, the ripples of thought stilled for the moment. With the conscious mind momentarily at rest, students are led toward creative imagery and are told to visualize, for example, a warm rich patch of earth.

"Feel the warmth of the sun, the life-giver of all things, beating down on this fertile bit of brown. Visualize a small sprout of plant life just breaking the surface of the ground. Continue to observe as the universal life force surges through the tiny plant urging it to reach for the heavens. As the plant grows, you will see leaves appearing on this creation of nature, and finally a bud forms, quivering with the urgency of life. Direct your consciousness to this swelling bud, as its petals begin to unfold one by one until finally the flower, a perfect red tulip, is completed. Imagine yourself so small that you can walk around inside this glorious creation, its inner structure assuming gigantic proportions as you look up at it. Now imagine yourself looking down on the tulip from above, going higher and higher until it disappears and your mind is again calm, peaceful, and blank."

This and similar mental exercises are extremely pleasant and play an integral part in developing the ability to visualize, to create mentally. As the conscious mind becomes calm and placid, the normal walls between the conscious mind and the subconscious become thinner, and the mind functions at increasingly lower levels—the levels of alpha and theta brain-wave frequencies, the levels of creative visualization, extrasensory perception, and in particularly sensitive individuals, the levels of hypnosis.

At these lower levels, for better or worse, the teacher whose mental lead you are following is programming you both verbally and nonverbally. In almost every class where these visualization sessions take place, there are students who are continually one step ahead of the instructor's voice. These supersensitive receiving stations believe they have anticipated the instructor's direction, but actually they have received the image through mind-to-mind contact.

We all assume that our thoughts are our own; frequently they are not. The mind can be compared to a radio, and those who are tuned in to the same station will hear or, in this case, think the same thing. Tuning in to the thoughts of those in your environment is unbelievably commonplace, particularly within the family structure, but this fact of mental gymnastics places an awesome responsibility on the yoga teacher to maintain a mental posture that is conscientiously constructive.

An experience of mine indicates how specific mind-to-mind contact can be. Aware that a person's thoughts are literally an open book to a sensitive or attuned person, I was considering the ways of protecting mental privacy when it is necessary. My husband and I were sitting in the living room, and I was thinking about, but not talking about, ways to accomplish "mind jamming," the blocking out of thought impulses in the presence of mental parasites. My husband was engrossed in a book, and I had just thought of the idea of mentally repeating the lines of "Mairzy Dotes," a nonsensical hit tune of the 1940s. As I was reviewing the lyrics in my mind, testing my memory of thirty years ago, Keith looked up and asked, "Do you know anything about the jamming of radio signals?"

As my students are stretched out on the floor in the relaxation period, I mentally repeat the following affirmation: "You are beautiful, God loves you, and I love you. All your thoughts, words, and actions are positive and constructive. You are perfectly healthy and have no self-destructive habits. Every day in every way you are getting better and better."

Should you prefer to learn yoga at home instead of joining a class, be sure to read the remainder of this chapter before attempting any of the postures. When you have read and understand the instructions, follow the Lesson Plan for Beginners outlined on page 84. Check with your doctor if you have any doubt about your physical ability to perform exercises.

Motivation

Some of you may be interested in yoga as a way to gain or lose weight or inches. Others may want to learn the secret of relaxation, and still others will be drawn by the mystic aura of meditation. All will find what they are seeking.

Motivation is the key to success in yoga. If your goal is physical perfection, visualize your desired physical goal. And you must keep your mind focused on this goal as you perform the postures, because that which you can visualize you can realize. Implanting a desirable image in your subconscious helps you produce this image in actuality.

Relaxation is probably the hardest aspect of yoga to teach yourself at home, simply because people tend not to take the time for it. Follow the instructions on page 185, and allow ten to fifteen minutes each day to really relax. After learning this technique, this state can be induced at will simply by using the mind to reconstruct the experience.

Meditation is the art of detuning physical and mental awareness so that you will have access to higher knowledge and awareness. If you are strongly drawn toward the meditation aspect of yoga, this is where your greatest gain will come. In short, wherever your greatest interest and highest motivation are, this is the area from which you will profit most.

You may be drawn to the relaxation aspect and find that a chronic sinus condition clears up mysteriously as well, because yoga is physical fitness with fringe benefits. Each posture has multiple benefits, and the entire body, internally and externally, will be improved.

Dress

Dress in loose, comfortable clothing that doesn't restrict your movements. Avoid garments that have zippers down the back, since these are uncomfortable in many postures. Never wear shoes while performing yoga.

Yoga movements require a flat surface with plenty of space to stretch out. Choose a well-ventilated spot where you can concentrate without being disturbed. Cover the surface of your practice area with a large towel, mat, or pad. Put this cover away after each exercise period, and use it only for yoga practice.

Do not practice yoga immediately after eating. It is advisable to wait ninety minutes after a light meal and three hours after a heavy meal.

Each posture has specific benefits, and you should know what the benefits of each one are. In this way you can best tailor a program to meet your particular needs. Remember to focus your concentration on what the posture is doing for you.

Rest Between Postures

Yoga postures are much less tiring than ordinary exercises, because you spend as much time resting between the postures as you do in performing them. Always lie down and wait until the muscles and the breathing are back to normal before proceeding to the next exercise. As you use a muscle, lactic acid, called the "acid of fatigue," is produced in the system, resulting in sore muscles and fatigue. Yoga's slow movements produce less lactic acid, and that which is generated is neutralized by the breathing and resting after each posture.

Start Slowly—Always Warm Up

A common mistake made by beginning as well as continuing students of yoga is not properly warming up the muscles before attempting the postures. Beginning students don't always realize how important it is, and continuing students are prone to feel, erroneously, that their general flexibility makes it unnecessary.

Yoga practice is generally done in the morning or at night, depending on individual schedules, and whether one is a day person or a night person. Those who prefer morning practice particularly need to include adequate warming-up exercises because the body stiffens up overnight. Morning stiffness is greatly reduced by taking a hot shower or bath prior to performing yoga.

There are several general warm-up exercises for the entire body, and there are some for specific areas. I recommend that my students begin the day with the elementary rocking exercise for loosening the spine (see page 88). And I suggest that the rocking be followed by four or five repetitions of suryanamaskar, the twelve-step Sun Salutation (page 90), which stretches all the muscles and ligaments in the body. Postures that require specific warm-ups will be so indicated on the page showing the posture and outlining instructions for it.

Progress is more important than perfection. A posture that is finally achieved after many failures, or one that has taken a long time to master, has more value than one effortlessly assumed. Any posture proving difficult is attempted three times during an exercise period and abandoned until the next day. This approach eliminates the frustration and pressure of our culture's demand for instant perfection. The sense of adequacy achieved when the posture is finally mastered is a step toward a more mature approach to life.

Always Stretch the Opposite Way

Yoga is a very balanced approach to physical fitness, and a posture that stretches your body in one direction must be followed by one that provides the opposite stretch. One way to make sure your home program remains balanced is to use the Basic Lesson Plan (page 84), add those for particular problem areas you want to work on, list the postures in the order that they should be performed, and then work through your list.

Practice Daily

Yoga practice begins slowly and takes into consideration the condition of the beginning student. Although its approach to physical fitness is gentle, yoga is progressive, and there are variations of each posture that will challenge even the most advanced student. As you become more advanced, mastering some of the postures that require additional strength, perform these more demanding postures early in your exercise period after the body is warmed up well but not yet fatigued.

The key to success in yoga is daily practice. According to the *Hatha Yoga Pradipika*, "Success is not obtained by wearing the dress of a yogi, nor by talking about it. Constant practice alone is the secret of success."

Use Your Own Internal Timer

One of Thoreau's best-known statements goes as follows: "If a man does not keep pace with his companions, perhaps it is because he hears a different drummer. Let him step to the music which he hears, however measured or far away."

On a purely philosophical plane this is another way of saying, "Do your own thing," be your own man, be yourself. From a practical, physical standpoint, this quote brings to mind the internal timer that we all have. If you've ever done exercises with an exercise program or been in a class and found yourself out of step with the group, this is your internal timer manifesting its presence.

Each person has his own internal rhythm, which is reflected in the rate of breathing, the speed of walking, and the general tempo of movements. With some people this is a slow and steady process; with others it is quick and erratic. When a yoga posture is to be held for a specific number of counts, count the number out to yourself, utilizing your own natural rhythm and timing.

As you progress, many of the postures will be maintained, or held motionless, for increasing intervals. This holding stretches blood vessels and directs the blood supply to a specific portion of the body.

Proportion

Not all bodies are proportioned alike. When I perform, for example, the Pose of Tranquillity (page 96), my body is in balance when the palms are positioned just above the knees as shown. The proper balance for you may be achieved by placing the palms anywhere from a point below the knees to considerably above the knees. Another good example of the problems posed by proportion is the Tripod, shown on page 114. This posture is absolutely impossible for anyone whose anatomical structure includes an unusually long femur, the bone that extends from the knee upward.

How Does Your Body "Give"?

Each body "gives" in a different direction, as the Standing Head-to-Knee Post on page 124 aptly illustrates. This posture appears to be the essence of simplicity, but performing it requires a degree of spinal flexibility that not all of us possess. This posture is more difficult for some people than other postures considered far more advanced. The same person who finds forward bending difficult will usually have little trouble bending backward. There is a natural inclination to avoid those postures most difficult for us. Keep in mind that the more a posture challenges you, the more your body needs it.

All those with normal bodies are born with sufficient flexibility to perform such postures easily. But over the years, we do not take advantage of our bodies' full range of movement, and we lose the ability to move as nature intended.

The Best Age for Yoga

There is no best age for yoga. Retirement-age students are filling yoga classes across the country, and there are experimental classes being conducted in preschool and nursery schools. The largest groups are those over thirty, but it will benefit all who participate.

The yoga path of self-realization can be compared to a lavish buffet that offers vast and varied types of nourishment. And as with a buffet, one can take as much or as little as is wanted or needed.

Those partaking of the entire feast become yogis, and yoga is their entire life, providing them with physical, mental, and spiritual sustenance. Others may select only that portion of yoga that will provide a firm, flexible, and well-functioning body. Some are comfortable only with those facets that lead to a well-disciplined and controlled mind. In any event, the yoga path will benefit all who travel it, regardless of the degree of their participation and commitment.

Even people who have no interest in a yoga program can be helped with specific physical problems. The Hand and Wrist Exercise shown on page 183 is helpful for anyone plagued by fingers or wrists that are stiffened or sore due to arthritis, strain, or the aging process. Used as a preventive, it provides strong, flexible hands and wrists. The excellent series of foot exercises on page 184 increases circulation in the lower extremities. When movement of either hands or feet is painful or impaired, all of life becomes more difficult.

Yoga for Children

Formal yoga training traditionally begins at the age of six, but even younger children can enjoy some of the asanas and the yoga relaxation. Children should never be forced to do yoga postures or allowed to adopt any postures that might harm their developing bodies.

The Headstand is prohibited for very young children, because the skull is too soft and the neck is not strong enough to support the body's weight. Also forbidden are the Plough, the Shoulder Stand, and all folding-up postures in which the chin is pressed into the neck and chest.

With proper guidance children practicing yoga learn self-control, discipline, and good habits. Habits develop from the time of birth, and they might just as well be good ones. Children in yoga learn good habits regarding food, breathing, and posture. They also develop a gracefulness and suppleness that lasts for a lifetime.

Yoga relaxation techniques can be used to good advantage by mothers with small children, particularly those who still nap—but not willingly. Sit by the child with eyes closed as he lies down. In a quiet, calm voice tell him, "Think about your toes. . . . Tell them to go to sleep. . . . Think about your legs. . . . Tell them to go to sleep." Continue this step-by-step procedure all the way up the back of the body and then down the front. Usually, the child will be asleep before you reach the end. Be sure to speak in a soft, slow voice, pausing a few seconds before shifting to another part of the body. This may take five minutes of your time, but it's worth it. You'll also be teaching your child the all-important art of relaxation.

Precautions

Just as aspirin is therapeutic in normal doses in normal people, but prohibited in special cases, so yoga must be approached cautiously by those with specific physical conditions. The inverted poses, such as the Headstand, Shoulder Stand, and Pose of Tranquillity, are some of the finest postures in yoga—except for anyone with a history of heart trouble, blood pressure over 150 or under 100, chronic nasal catarrh, constipation, running ears or pus in the ears, or weak eye capillaries. Many people with undetected weak eye capillaries discover this only when inverted postures cause bloodshot eyes.

Leg-raising exercises are great for the abdominal muscles but play havoc with weak lower backs. People with this problem should place their hands or a small pillow under the small of the back for support while doing leg raises. Yoga is helpful for back problems caused by lack of exercise, but persons with back problems induced by a herniated disk require medical direction in formulating an exercise plan.

Older people, even those without known medical complications, must use a very gentle and gradual approach to some postures, particularly those that require the body to be bent backward. As a person ages, unless physical exercise has been a consistent part of one's life, the disks that provide cushioning between vertebrae deteriorate, their ability to provide the necessary cushioning is lessened, and they become greatly more susceptible to rupture.

Yoga vs. Calisthenics

Many of the postures or exercises utilized in yoga look to the novice very much like exercises found in any physical exercise or calisthenics class. There are differences, however, differences that account for yoga's staying power in contrast to the rise and decline of other systems at the dictates of a fickle public fancy.

The most important difference is that in gymnastics the mind remains uninvolved, whereas in yoga the mind is of great importance. In each posture the mind must concentrate on the benefits of that posture. You must visualize your body as you want it to be and concentrate on this image.

Still another difference is the speed with which exercises and postures are performed. In gymnastics the repetitions are performed quickly, involving violent muscular movements. When the body is moved rapidly, momentum carries it to the point of pain, and beyond the point of pain, at such a speed that injury often results. In yoga all movements are slow and rhythmic, the point of pain being approached so gradually that motion can be halted before it becomes uncomfortable.

In calisthenics breathing is not an essential part of the exercise; in yoga each exercise is coupled with specific inhalation, holding of the breath, and exhalation. This breathing calms the nervous system and neutralizes the fatiguing lactic acid produced by muscular movements, but most important, it increases prana in the system and directs it to specific parts of the body.

Yoga is the only system that teaches discipline through immobility. As mentioned earlier, the word "yoga" means union or to join. In holding a posture for two, three, or even five minutes, a subtle joining of mind and body takes place. It is something that must be experienced to be believed. The holding of postures provides a better understanding of how your body reacts under pressure. And there is a serenity that comes with the uniting of mind and body in a concentrated effort. From a physical standpoint the holding of postures stretches blood vessels and directs the blood supply to a specific portion of the body.

Whereas calisthenics and gymnastics are concerned with only the muscular structure of the body, yoga encompasses the entire human organism. All of the systems of the body—the muscular structure, the nervous system, the digestive system, the elimination system, the respiratory system, and the endocrine system—are beneficially involved in the practice of yoga.

The Endocrine System

One of the most amazing facets of yoga is its thorough acquaintance with the workings of the endocrine system. It is amazing because yoga is centuries old, and knowledge of the endocrine system has been a part of the medical profession as we know it since only 1899.

While the yogis of antiquity did not know, for example, that the thyroid gland is situated in the neck, they were cognizant of the various glandular regions. Yoga literature is the first place these glandular regions were mentioned. And these ancient writings also recognized that the glandular regions exerted far-reaching effects on the entire human organism.

The endocrine system consists of ductless glands that manufacture various hormones and secrete them directly into the bloodstream. Tiny quantities of these hormones have powerful effects on the body. A healthy and normally functioning endocrine system is vital, influencing our appearance, disposition, moods, and behavior. It also affects growth, the shape of the body, and the way in which the body uses food.

The person whose endocrine system is in good working order is usually strong, vigorous, optimistic, mentally alert, and generally happy. An improperly functioning endocrine system can produce obesity, timidity, moroseness, fear, depression, ovarian disturbances, loss of virility, and arrested mental and physical development in children.

While the endocrine system is out of balance, it is generally a functional disorder rather than an organic one. This means that the glands are healthy, but they are receiving an inadequate supply of nerve energy due to undernourishment. This undernourishment is the result of an improperly oxygenated bloodstream.

Yoga exercises and breathing keep the glands healthy and functioning properly. There are specific postures to stimulate each of the various endocrine glands, but a balanced yoga program is usually sufficient to maintain a healthy endocrine system.

The pituitary gland, which looks like a cherry dangling from the base of the brain, has been called the master gland. It secretes several hormones, which regulate the growth of the entire body and the development and function of the sex glands, and influence other endocrine glands. The Headstand and other inverted postures stimulate the pituitary gland.

The pineal is located in the upper rear portion, and between the halves, of the brain. The function of the pineal is still a mystery to the medical profession. In 1958 researchers isolated a substance secreted by the pineal and named it melatonin. Yogis believe the pineal is the seat of intuition, or ESP, and is connected with occult powers. René Descartes, the seventeenth-century French philosopher, believed it was the dwelling place of the soul.

Many scientists claim that in our prehistoric ancestors it was a third eye. It, too, is stimulated by the Headstand and other inverted postures. These inverted postures are believed to increase intuitive powers by augmenting the nourishing flow of blood to the pineal gland.

The thyroid gland, located in the neck, produces the hormone thyroxine, which regulates metabolism. Metabolism determines the rate at which the body uses food and oxygen. A sluggish thyroid gland slows a person down physically and mentally. The skin becomes coarse, the person gains weight, and the mind loses its alertness. The Shoulder Stand is the most effective posture to stimulate the thyroid and is of particular benefit for overweight persons.

The parathyroids are four tiny glands located on the back surface of the thyroid gland. These glands produce parathormone, which regulates the way the body uses calcium and phosphorus. Insufficient parathormone causes the calcium level in the body to drop while the amount of phosphorus rises. This causes muscle twitching and possibly convulsions. The Shoulder Stand helps maintain the parathyroid glands in good working order.

The thymus gland, located in the chest, is another gland that baffles the medical profession. Its exact function has never been determined, but since it becomes small and inactive at puberty, it is thought to be related to growth and development in children.

The adrenal glands are located above each kidney and produce several hormones, the most notable of which is adrenaline. When a person is angry or frightened, it is the adrenaline pouring into the bloodstream that prepares him to fight or run away. The heart beats faster, blood pressure rises, and the bronchial tubes dilate to allow the person to breathe more quickly and easily. The pupils of the eyes enlarge to admit more light, and the liver releases more sugar into the bloodstream to provide increased energy. The functions controlled by the adrenal's hormones are vital.

The sex glands located in the pelvic region control reproduction and are intimately involved in the development of female characteristics in women and male characteristics in men. Many yoga postures contribute to the good health of the sex glands.

The yogis of old knew intuitively that their postures and exercises had far-reaching effects on the entire human organism. Twentieth-century yogis have the added reassurance that these ancient concepts are now reinforced by medical facts.

One of the reasons yoga has maintained its aura of mystery is that its devotees frequently exhibit increased awareness or expanded consciousness—in other words, ESP. Some authorities attribute this to the yoga postures, fasting, and autosuggestion. Another possible explanation for these heightened psychic faculties relates to yoga's involvement of the endocrine system.

Yoga as Ecology

Are you often exhausted without any discernible reason, emotionally drained, or nervous and irritable? Perhaps you have neglected to think of ecology in terms of yourself. Yoga is a form of ecology, but ecology in the most personal sense. Ecology experts are concerned with our larger planetary environment; yogis concentrate on the individual environment— the human body, mind, and spirit.

Environmentalists are concerned with our squandering of the earth's natural resources, while the yogi is concerned with the squandering of the individual's life force. Energy or life force is generated through the stretching and breathing exercises of yoga and should be used for self-development.

To preserve vital life force, try to eliminate nervous habits, avoid negative persons and idle chatter, and do not overstimulate the senses. How many people around you are tapping their feet, twisting their hair, biting their fingernails, chain smoking, chewing gum, or gesturing expansively? These nervous habits, many of which are expressions of fear, anger, or anxiety, waste vital energy. They leave people feeling nervous, jittery, and up in the air.

The yoga doctrine, and some of the greatest thinkers of the literary world, place great value on the quality of silence. On this subject Henry Wadsworth Longfellow said: "The silence of the place was like a sleep, so full of rest it seemed." Noise-pollution experts, a century later, are proving the wisdom of this observation. And Emerson, in true yogic fashion, commented, "Let us be silent that we may hear the whispers of the gods."

Nowhere in the world has the effect of the human voice been studied so thoroughly as in India. Every spoken word there is regarded as falling into one of three categories: creation, preservation, or destruction. This same categorization might apply to all actions of the world population in the monumental task of righting our planetary environment.

Kinds of Postures—and the Reasons for Them

Yogic wisdom was not impeded in its search for the nature of man by our current trend toward specialization. The sages who set up this system of human development saw man as an integrated whole, not merely a skeletal structure, a network of nerve endings, a pumping station, or a complex computer. They also realized that the whole was far greater than the sum of its parts. A human being is like a gigantic jigsaw puzzle with thousands of pieces. Each has its own place, and should any segment be missing or out of place, the picture of man is neither true nor complete.

Medical science and the facts of evolution support the theory that those parts of the human body that are not used eventually atrophy and are lost. Anyone who has had a leg or an arm in a cast knows that even a short period of inactivity reduces the size and strength of the muscles involved. When a cast is removed from a broken leg, that leg is much smaller and weaker because the muscles have been immobilized. Scientists caution us that the current decline in walking will eventually produce a humanoid species whose legs are incapable of bearing and transporting the weight of the body.

The human body should be moved in every way that is capable of motion, and the postures of hatha-yoga provide a full range of motion for the entire organism. The various types of asanas and the reasons they are important in a well-rounded program are covered later in this chapter. Because most yoga postures have multiple benefits, there is some overlapping.

Effects of Stunted Nervous Systems

Yoga's concept of the complex interaction of the human system has been reinforced by the research of Dr. Glenn Doman and Dr. Carl Delacato, pioneers in the growing field of learning disabilities in children. Their research has greatly increased medical knowledge concerning the connection between the use of the eyes and hands and the development of the brain and nervous system.

Men have walked on the surface of the moon, and yet there are still Stone Age tribes—the Kingu, Caraja, and Kalapalo—deep in the jungles of the Amazon that are among the most primitive people in existence. They have no system of writing or numbering, they do not use metal, and their large primitive huts have no floors.

This absence of floors held great theoretical significance for Delacato and Doman. Babies must learn to crawl before they walk in order to achieve full neurological development. Children who are not permitted to crawl, whether because of snakes, insects, or even an overindulgent mother, will grow up underdeveloped. Doman and Delacato's findings in investigating these primitive tribes are related in Dr. Delacato's book, *A New Start for the Child with Reading Problems*, from which I quote as follows:

We searched everywhere for babies on the ground, but could find none. At each village we offered to pay mothers to place their up-to-18-months-old babies on the ground, but they refused.

We tested many children of all ages for general neurological fitness and we found that, as a group, they were seriously lacking in nervous system development. We found that they had difficulty in using their two eyes together; their creeping was extremely awkward, and very few of the group had developed sidedness (a dominant hand, eye or foot).

They did not pass our tests for the development of the nervous system; in fact most of them performed as poorly on our tests as did . . . American children with reading problems.

The human brain and nervous system develop through use. A baby must learn to use both eyes together. Initially, infants use one eye at a time; as they learn to crawl and coordinate one hand with the opposite knee, the head is up from the floor, and both eyes begin working together. Children who are always carried, or those who, for any reason, do not crawl and creep, develop stunted nervous systems.

By its second birthday a baby has developed sidedness—one hand, one foot, one eye becomes dominant. Of all the earth's creatures only man has this sidedness, and only man possesses language and speech. These two facts are definitely related. Dr. Delacato continues:

If the left half of the brain becomes dominant, the child becomes right-handed. . . . The dominant half of the brain becomes the language center. Here is where reading and decoding of speech takes place, as well as the storage of language. If one of the halves does not become dominant, then the brain is not completely developed and a problem with reading usually results.

In addition to reading difficulties, there are frequently personality and behavioral problems related to lack of sidedness, further proof that man is an integrated entity. Dr. Paul Dunn, director of Children's Therapeutic Programs in Oak Park, Illinois, explains that "this is because such neurologically deprived children use up such great amounts of emotional energy just trying to read, to work with numbers, and to coordinate their bodies that there is nothing left for personality development." These children are frequently irritable, hyperactive, uncoordinated, and unusually thin, though many eat ravenously.

A method of treating these children has been developed, known as Doman-Delacato "patterning," in which older children creep and crawl as if they were babies, filling in, albeit belatedly, the gaps in their neurological development. In this patterning it is actually the eyes that are being trained to coordinate with the motions of the hands while crawling and creeping. This may sound like witchcraft to the uninitiated, and the method is admittedly controversial in medical and educational circles, but I have closely observed a youngster treated by means of this method, and the results were nothing short of miraculous. In the words of that child: "I used to try so hard to do things right, to get good grades in school, and to cooperate at home, and it didn't work. Everybody was always mad at me. Now I don't even have to try, and everything is going right for me."

Eye and Neck Exercises

The eyes have inspired poets and lovers since time began. And no one underestimates their practical value in leading us through life. Few, however, outside the Doman-Delacato circles, realize that their ability to move together smoothly is indicative of sound neurological development. If the eye exercises in this book are difficult for you, may I suggest that you read Dr. Delacato's *A New Start for the Child with Reading Problems* for more insight into this problem.

Even people who exercise regularly frequently forget that the body has a head and a neck. The neck is capable of such a degree of motion that it is possible to look behind you without turning the body at all. Lack of adequate use makes the neck a primary target for premature aging. If performing neck rolls conjures up images of the gravel pit, the aging process has set in regardless of the date on your birth certificate. The gritty, gravelly sound that you hear is crepitation, a by-product of aging, which will be eliminated through regular practice of the neck rolls.

The neck and shoulder areas are also tension magnets. Each time you are interrupted by a phone call, the cry of a child, or collide with any other of life's irritants, your shoulder blades tighten, and the shoulders raise slightly. As the day progresses, more tension builds up in this area causing pain in the back of the neck, achy shoulders, and headaches. This tightness will not go away automatically but will be eliminated by the neck exercises. If the neck rolls leave you feeling drowsy, it's relief of tension that you feel.

Spinal Flexing Exercises

There is an axiom in yoga that you are as old as your spine is flexible. Another basic premise is that age relates to one's ability to change more than the condition of one's actual chronological age. Quite simply, age is inflexibility—mental or physical. Of the two, an inflexible mind is far more indicative of old age than a stiff body. When the mind is incapable of viewing situations in a new light, or accepting the value of new concepts, the aging process has set in.

The spine, as the spinal column or vertebral column is commonly called, is an anatomical architectural marvel. At birth there are thirty-three bones, called vertebrae, in the spine, some of which fuse during the growth years to provide an adult vertebral count of twenty-four. The normal adult spine contains four gentle curves, nature's protection against jarring and the resultant injury to the spinal cord it encases and the brain. The spinal cord extends from the lower part of the brain through the bony arches formed in each vertebra. Between each vertebra a pair of nerves branches off, messengers carrying out the complex communication system between the brain and all parts of the body. Spinal flexing exercises benefit the entire body by maintaining a tension-free spine, assuring safe passage for life's mighty couriers.

The rapport that exists between the human body and the human mind shows up dramatically here, for as the spine grows increasingly flexible, the mind also sheds its rigidity. The physical performance of a posture deemed impossible forces a wedge in the closed mind, a wedge that opens wider with each new accomplishment.

Man being the only animal with a vertical spine is spiritually significant. Yoga views man's spine as a spiritual link between heaven and earth, between God and man.

The Inverted Postures

The quest for eternal youth has always been a popular crusade, and Ponce de Leon might have been more successful had he kicked up his heels a bit more often, or at least gotten his feet higher than his head on a regular basis. Far from being frivolous, these inverted postures have almost a miraculous way of slowing the sands of time and the aging process.

Two of the most devastating symptoms of aging are the onset of wrinkles and the loss of the moist, youthful complexion so synonymous with youth. Both of these symptoms result from the fact that, with increasing age, the pull of gravity deprives the facial area of adequate circulation. The slant board, that favorite of the Hollywood set, reflects the correlation between adequate circulation to the face and the maintenance of a youthful appearance.

Lack of circulation in the face and head also is responsible for much of the lessening of mental acuity associated with aging. The brain requires a monumentally disproportionate share—7 percent—of the body's blood supply. The vital needs of the average man make it necessary for the heart to pump a pint and a half of blood every minute to the brain; women require less because they're smaller. The steady practice of inverted postures improves memory by increasing circulation to the brain.

Mastery of the Headstand, called the king of asanas, has an elevating effect on one's confidence and self-esteem. Though it is not difficult physically, many Westerners at first mentally underestimate their ability to do it and are inclined to rate its eventual performance as a tremendous accomplishment.

Yoga increases spiritual awareness and so-called extrasensory perception, it is believed, by reason of the extra blood supply directed to the pineal gland during the practice of these inverted postures.

Stretching Postures

Stretching postures mold the body into pleasing lines of symmetry. Not only do they feel good, but most important, they relieve the body and mind of its accumulations of tension.

Tension and irritation can, quite literally, give you a pain in the neck. They can, in fact, give you a pain in any area of the body in which muscles are continually subjected to tension without release and relaxation. Medical experiments demonstrate that repeated tensing of a muscle without its subsequent relaxation results in loss of length of that muscle. Then, when that muscle is suddenly required to stretch, it cannot do so properly and reacts by going into spasm or by tearing. Yoga postures and exercises are specifically designed to stretch and relax tense areas of the body before they become serious problems.

Some areas of the body are particularly prone to stiffening up even with regular exercise. Two such areas are the hamstrings (the tendons located at the back of the knees) and the lower back. One of the most effective exercises for these areas is the Sitting Five-Step, which is shown on page 120.

Balance Postures

One of the hallmarks of an emotionally stable person is a deep and abiding interest in something other than self. Many people make the mistake of directing all their interest toward one subject—business, family, fun—and risk becoming one-dimensional. These people lack insight into one important fact of life—the intrinsic value of maintaining a proper balance in all activities.

Little in the universe can long endure without balance. Its significance is

easily understood in the financial area, but consider also its value in
nature, nations, and nutrition. Balance is vital in the world of fashion, and
those suffering from mental disturbances are said to be "unbalanced." Any
relationship between people or countries that gets out of balance is headed
for trouble. And in the rearing of children, parents strive for a good balance of love and discipline.

Realizing the subtle connection between mind and body, many yoga
postures train the body in the art of balance. These postures are doubly
valuable because they aid in developing not only a sense of physical balance but also mental equilibrium and tranquillity. The physical effort of
balancing the body is reflected on the mind's nervous system. Many students who experience no trouble with the "brute strength" postures find
balancing postures difficult, perhaps a subconscious reminder of the need
for balance—physically, mentally, and spiritually.

A pointer that makes balance postures easier may seem strange until
you try it. Pick out a solid vertical object, and rivet your attention to it
while attempting these postures. This could be a doorframe, a post, or
any other solid upright object. While gazing on this object, assume that
you have its balance and stability.

The current enthusiasm for yoga in the United States in some ways
threatens to create an unhealthy imbalance in the minds of many devotees.
Although the mental and physical discipline inherent in yoga practice is
greatly beneficial, it does not necessarily follow that Western technological
advances are all bad. Just as the Western world has much to learn from
the spiritual and mystical East, there is much that the West can teach, too.
Neither hemisphere has an absolute monopoly on wisdom or truth.

Western civilization has been called sick, but neither is the East an ideal
example. What is needed seems to be a mixture of the two—a blending
of Oriental spirituality and mysticism and Western practicality. The Orient
has shown a lack of competence in dealing with the external environment
of man, and the Occident has shown a similar void in developing man's
inner nature.

Twisting Postures

It is a well-known fact that not many human beings realize their inherent
potential. This generally refers to mental capacities, but it is equally true
in the realm of the physical.

The human spine is capable of a corkscrew twisting motion, but very
few of our daily activities provide this form of movement. Since areas of
mobility that are not used are lost, it is essential to include some form of
exercise that will laterally twist the spine. Besides providing a powerful

stretch for the back muscles, they realign minor vertebral irregularities and ease tension throughout the spine.

Many of the twisting postures are complicated, making it necessary to follow the step-by-step directions with extreme care. For this reason they are useful in training the mind to concentrate. The spine houses the seven main chakras, which are fully explained later in this chapter, giving it a specific spiritual significance.

Exercises for Hands and Feet

The hands and feet, our tools of accomplishment and locomotion, deserve more attention than they get. Swelling of both is commonplace, and though there can be many reasons for this phenomenon, a common one is loss of muscle tone. Blood circulation depends upon cooperation between the heart, which pumps the blood, and the muscles. As the muscles move, they squeeze blood vessels and aid circulation. When muscles do not move, because of inactivity or because they are unable to, such as after a stroke, congestion results, and abnormal amounts of fluid accumulate in the tissues causing swelling.

Reflexology is a method of therapy based on massage of the reflexes in the hands and feet. Every part of the human body has a corresponding reflex in the palms of the hands and on the bottoms of the feet. Physical malfunctioning of any part of the body produces a tiny but painful crystal in the foot reflex linked with that part of the body that has gone awry. These crystals cause congestion, slowing the flow of blood to the afflicted part of the body. A system of massage breaks down these tiny crystals, restoring proper circulation, and reportedly leads to healing of the physical disorder.

Civilization may have done great things for the rest of the body, but the foot has been shortchanged. Prehistoric man, who walked barefoot over all sorts of terrain, had a style of life that provided adequate foot massage, and consequently there was no need for foot reflexology.

Mothers who are eager to see their babies walk at the earliest possible age are quick to encase little feet in hard-sole shoes to speed up the process. Children of any age usually kick off their shoes the minute they hit the front door, and their intuition is sound in this case. Even Dr. Spock recommends shoes only as a necessity for protection from cold and hazardous objects, because he believes that feet and leg muscles develop better without them.

Shoes, which restrict normal foot movement, as well as the aging process tend to reduce circulation in the feet. People of any age will be amazed at the obvious increased circulation provided by the series of foot exercises on page 184. Surprisingly pleasant for everyone, these exercises are especially beneficial to the elderly and can be performed with the help of someone else if necessary.

Life becomes more difficult when movement of either hands or feet is painful. The hand exercises shown on page 183 provide an excellent way to maintain the hands in good health, though normal daily use provides its own form of reflexology for the hands. These exercises are particularly effective for stiff or sore wrists and generally aid discomfort from arthritis, injury, or aging. The wearing of women's stretch gloves, either nylon knit or nylon-Spandex, also eases morning arthritic stiffness. According to one survey, fifty-three of fifty-six patients showed improvement when such gloves were worn overnight.

Meditative Postures

Four of yoga's postures are meditative—the Lotus, the pose of an adept, the Ankle Lock Pose, and the Easy Pose. The remainder of the asanas are called cultural postures. Meditative postures physically stretch the knees, thigh joints, and ankles, but their primary purpose is to firmly anchor the lower body so that there is no chance of toppling over during meditation. These postures assure that the spine, the spiritual link between heaven and earth, remains straight. Prolonged immobility in these postures slows down the metabolic processes, and the mind concentrates with ease, freed from the distractions of physiological rumblings.

Relaxation

Ask anyone what he or she does for relaxation, and the answers are likely to range through such active pursuits as swimming, horseback riding, skiing, scuba diving, dancing, sewing, antiquing, and gardening. The more sedentary types will say they relax by reading, watching television, collecting stamps, painting oils, and so on. All these things are great. But they are forms of recreation, not relaxation.

Another misconception is that relaxation is a condition automatically produced by flopping into a chair or onto a couch or a bed. One of the reasons Americans have so much trouble relaxing is that they don't have any real conception of the true nature of relaxation. They assume it is a passive process that just happens; actually, it is an active process that you cause to happen, and it is your mind that calls the shots in this all-important state. Follow the instructions on page 185, and be sure to include the relaxation each day following practice of the asanas.

Occasionally a student will come to me after the second or third class and express concern that more attention has not been given to mental control. Beginning students are told of the subtle rapport that exists between the body and mind, but some find it difficult to understand that they must learn to control the body first. As the body yields to the direction of the mind, it is paving the way for the mind-controlling exercises that follow.

Yoga's Effect on Aging

We all start aging at birth, and each body has its own set pattern of aging. One major objective of yoga postures is to reverse this aging process by strengthening your weakest muscles. A posture that is particularly difficult for you to achieve indicates that the muscles involved need strengthening. The human aging process can aptly be compared to centrifugal force— a body in motion tends to remain in motion, and a body at rest tends to remain at rest.

Your body's rhythmic pattern of aging has been long established, and exercises that challenge and disrupt that pattern will not be particularly pleasant for you. When you encounter such an exercise, master your muscles—don't let them master you. Once your aging pattern has been slowed down, stopped, and reversed, these postures will no longer prove formidable, and your entire system will show signs of rejuvenation and youth.

However, be prepared for these stumbling blocks. Your body will resist your efforts to change its rhythm of aging; there will be times when the effort seems disproportionate to the promised gain, but if you stick with it, the rewards will surprise you.

The Causes of Aging

The aging process has been called a series of small collapses and is thought to be inevitable, but need it be? The Hunzas of the Himalayas defy all the known concepts of aging. Nestled in a nearly inaccessible remote valley, the thirty thousand inhabitants of Hunzaland may have been the inspiration for Shangri-La, where the life expectancy far exceeds the biblical threescore and ten, where the elders still engage in hard physical labor as well as play, outwitting the physical diseases and mental decline thought in this country to be synonymous with aging. Divorce, juvenile delinquency, crime, and disease—human, plant, or animal—are unknown to the Hunzakuts. Although their active longevity has mystified the world for some two thousand years, their lives strikingly correlate with yoga teachings.

The tiny state of Hunza is an agricultural community, one that is not mechanized, and each step in food production is done manually. The labor involved in tilling the hilly terrain provides vigorous physical activity for all the Hunzakuts from children to elders. Their physical labors are balanced with equally vigorous recreational games—volleyball, archery, polo, and tennis.

Their diet is yogalike, consisting mainly of whole-grain products, leafy vegetables, fruits, dairy products, and very little meat. Though the Hunzas are not vegetarians, meat is sparse, and what is available is prepared in stews to make it go further. Vegetables are not sprayed with chemicals, but are prepared immediately after picking to preserve the vitamins and minerals. Cooking time is very short and done with little water, to conserve nutritional quality, and the cooking liquid is also served. A staple of the Hunza diet is chapatti, a whole-grain unleavened bread, which is vastly superior to the refined, devitalized, nutritionless white bread so commonplace on American tables.

Fresh fruits are eaten raw with the skin intact. This is an important factor because the skin of fresh fruits is a rich source of minerals that are lost in peeling, cooking, or even zealous scrubbing. Hunza milk is unpasteurized, and the only oil in their diet is a polyunsaturated one that is extracted from the kernels of apricots. Significantly, Hunzas do not suffer from heart attacks, strokes, or circulatory disease.

Fasting, an observance of many yogis, is a matter of necessity with the Hunzas. Their food supply is often depleted during the long winter months and cannot be replenished until a new crop is grown. During this time they manage to survive on water provided by the melting of glacier snow, a grayish, gritty substance that provides a rich daily supply of the minerals that cannot be stored in the body.

Competition is unknown in this agricultural village, where prayer and meditation are part of the daily regime. There are no environmental stressors such as noise, pollution, or chemical food additives. Stress depletes the human system of its B vitamins, so necessary in a sound nervous system. Though many of the body's cells regenerate themselves, this seems not to apply to nerve cells. Perhaps one of the Hunzakuts' mainstays, then, is the sound nervous system derived from their diet and stressless life-style.

The Hunzakuts are the antithesis of our youth-driven culture, perhaps because they have found the Land of Eternal Youth. No one in their culture dreads old age. The people believe that a person is as old as he feels, looks, and behaves. Their lack of fear regarding aging underscores a spiritual law—the law of attraction—which postulates that whatever the mind dwells on, whether good or bad, the mind attracts. The Hunzakuts' total lack of fear is undoubtedly significant in their extraordinary lives.

Much of the Hunzas' way of life is impossible to duplicate in urban America. This example is used only to illustrate that time is not the only enemy to be considered in fighting undue and premature aging. The pull of central gravity on the body's organs and lack of circulation in the face and head, as described in Chapter 1, are also factors. So, also, are too much stress, incorrect breathing, too little sleep, apathy, tension, improper eating habits, and lack of exercise. Another contributor to the aging process that receives too little attention is loss of vitality, the loss of an abiding interest in life.

My ninety-two-year-old father-in-law, who practiced law until the age of ninety, commented recently that the joys of old age are highly overrated. He made this comment not as a complaint, but with the same humor that has characterized his life. During this same visit he held the family spellbound with his rendition of Emerson's "Self-Reliance" and passages from Shakespeare, long ago committed to memory and faultlessly recalled these many years later. My husband affectionately suggests that his father's Welsh ancestry carries a built-in love of the dramatic, particularly when the Welshman is center stage surrounded by an attentive audience. This may be part of the answer, but more important, even ninety-two years has not squelched his zest for life and vital energy.

And Indra Devi, who was born in 1899, is another living reprimand for those who start most conversations with "I just don't have the energy I used to have," or "I seem to have lost interest," or "I just can't be bothered any more." Indra Devi moves with the fluid grace of a teen-ager, effortlessly folds her legs in Lotus Posture while standing on her head, and meets each new day with an enthusiasm that is ageless. Those who use the middle years as a justification for not living life to the fullest are marked by the greatest ager of all—a loss of vital energy and enthusiasm. When these are gone, the body lacks animation and appears old, regardless of chronological age.

To maintain vital energy, you must cultivate a positive mental attitude. View each passing year as an opportunity to learn something new, to meet new people, and to help someone. It is standard therapy for the bereaved widow to get involved in helping at an orphanage or to occupy part of her time in charity work or some other endeavor that will redirect her interests outside herself and her own grief. Although losing a mate is one of life's severest traumas, meeting it maturely does provide the stimulus for a broadening of interests, and thus it becomes an antidote to aging.

Practical Applications of Yoga

Western applications of yoga are characteristic of the basic difference between the Eastern mind and the Western mind. When Eastern man finds something worthwhile and of intrinsic value, he absorbs it, contemplates it, and savors it. Western man, on the other hand, is more geared to putting worthy innovations to practical use. In our culture yoga should not be regarded merely as a pleasant form of physical fitness and mental stability. Yoga should be regarded as a tool for living.

The chapter on breathing explained the tranquilizing effect of yoga breathing, but the asanas have practical applications also. Skiing is one of the fastest-growing sports in the United States, and each fall newspapers and magazines urge skiers to get their legs in shape before taking to the slopes. The yoga leg exercises are excellent ski conditioners, because they increase ·strength and pliability in legs and ankles and improve balance. Equestrians will also find the leg exercises, and the balance postures, useful in horseback riding.

In the area of sports, probably the most mental game in the world is golf, which teams up physical coordination and mental concentration. Beginning golfers often thrill to their occasional perfect shot, but to score well consistently, golfers must know the elements of each shot and be able to visualize them mentally. That which you can visualize you can create in actual experience. The first time my score totaled less than 100 for eighteen holes was actually done as an experiment to see if yoga methods could advantageously be applied to golf.

I know the elements of the game and what constitutes a proper shot, but I was guilty of the common tendency to get too much right hand into my swing. Golfers will recognize this as "killing the ball"—trying too hard for distance. In this experiment I concentrated on keeping my mental attention riveted to a spot approximately two inches below the elbow on top of the left forearm. Each time my concentration remained there, instead of on the right hand, the shot was perfect, the ball going much farther than when I consciously tried to hit a long shot. On the green lack of practice has ruined many a promising game, and the game in question was my second of the season. Before each putt I mentally rehearsed the shot, visualizing the ball dropping into the cup. I completely eliminated three-putt greens, the nemesis of the weekend golfer, and came in with a total of thirty-three putts for eighteen holes.

To be of any statistical value, this sort of experiment would have to be repeated a number of times with greater numbers of people who had established handicaps to see if their handicaps could, indeed, be lowered. The results would be interesting, and if they pointed in the direction I think they would, undoubtedly would lure more men into yoga classes.

Even discussing a recreational pursuit in connection with yoga may seem a sacrilege to serious devotees, but to do the most good, yoga must be an integral part of one's life, and it need not be heavy and sanctimonious. A mature approach to life must reflect balance, and a life devoted entirely to the contemplation of one's navel, an erroneous concept of yoga, would be clearly out of balance—and dull.

Healing Aspects of Yoga

No reputable yoga teacher will ever tell a student that yoga will cure anything. When cures for specific or chronic ailments occur, it is because the entire body as a whole reaches a new high level of efficiency, and healing takes place spontaneously. Hippocrates, the father of medicine, told his Greek disciples some twenty-four centuries ago that disease is not only suffering but also toil. This toil is the body's fight to regain health. He recognized the healing force of nature that cures from within.

Overzealous students of yoga, who underestimate the body's tremendous latent power of healing, often credit yoga with cures of everything from chronic diarrhea to gray hair. The body actually cures itself, and yoga is merely the catalyst that activates the healing power we all possess.

One of my students, a grandmother in her early fifties, many years ago suffered an accident to her left knee that destroyed the reflex action. Her doctor advised her that the damage was permanent and irreversible. This woman submits to an annual physical examination, and after two years of regular yoga practice, both she and her doctor were amazed to discover that the left knee reflex had been restored to perfect normalcy. The doctor maintains that this is the first such case he has witnessed; the woman gives full credit to yoga.

Another woman, whose forty-odd years had been plagued with asthma attacks, thought yoga might help her condition. She joined a class taught by a young teacher, one who lacked the experience of working with students who do not achieve the postures easily. This woman considered herself a complete failure in yoga, and yoga a failure in helping her asthma. She signed up for my class as a last resort. Thanks to the techniques I learned from Indra Devi, this woman soon mastered the postures, and even more important, the breathing that had previously defeated her. Her confidence grew, and her asthma attacks occurred less and less frequently.

Millions of people suffer from asthma, a disease characterized by wheezing, coughing, and difficulty in breathing. Yoga postures and breathing exercises help many of these people. Although breathing is an automatic process, yoga teaches an awareness of the breathing process and how to control it. Asthma sufferers who learn controlled yoga breathing are often able to duplicate this control when threatened with an attack. Yoga breathing also helps control the nerves and emotions, long known to complicate the problems of asthmatics.

Variations of the Fish posture (pages 101–104) remove stiffness from the cervical spine and increase circulation in this area. This helps reduce spasms in the bronchial area which plague asthmatics.

Another student, scheduled for varicose-vein surgery, avoided it when her veins surprisingly became normal; another has eliminated debilitating migraine headaches; and still another has gone back to skiing after being sidelined for years with arthritis. These success stories go on and on, and make the teaching of yoga a supremely satisfying experience. When the human body, mind, and spirit work together in health and harmony, the results are nothing short of miraculous.

Yoga also builds inner resources—that extra something that allows those who have it to meet the adversities of life without being crushed by them. We have all come to associate this grace under pressure with the Kennedy clan. Internal resources, too, are physical, mental, and spiritual. Faith, that basic trust in and acceptance of the dictates of a Higher Power, is a spiritual resource. A positive mental attitude is the greatest mental internal resource one can have. Even though you cannot control everything that happens to you, you can control how you react to these events. The courage to view each defeat or disappointment in life as an avenue of growth, as an incentive to adapt to the inevitability of change, provides an inner resilience that separates the winners from the losers.

Physical inner resources are most dramatically demonstrated by professional athletes and Olympic competitors who have honed their physical skills to an almost unbelievably fine edge. The lack of inner physical strength is the unsuspected culprit in many of man's ills. Weak abdominal muscles that permit the abdomen to sag place a strain on the back and are often the cause of low-back pain. Victims of such backaches are often surprised by their doctor's advice to perform exercises to strengthen the abdominal muscles. This same principle is the reason expectant mothers frequently suffer from low-back pain.

Many of today's back ills can be traced to the era when teen-age girls took to girdles along with their first pair of nylons. Girdle-wearing resulted in their dependence on external supports instead of developing inner resources—in this case, abdominal muscles. The classic yoga Headstand from a postural standpoint is the greatest developer of internal resources. It involves nearly all of the muscles in the body and instills a tremendous sense of self-confidence, a necessary first step in developing a positive mental attitude.

The Symbolism of Yoga

A symbol is a sign that stands for some object or an idea. Each country has a national flag that symbolizes "my country." Every religion utilizes symbols, the cross being that of Christianity. The ship was an early Christian symbol that represented the Church, in which the "faithful are carried over the sea of life."

Yoga, too, has its symbols. The Lotus posture shown on page 112 is the universal symbol of yoga. It is named after the lotus plant, the national flower of India. The lotus is a variety of water lily that originates in the mud, grows on a weak stalk through the water, and blooms on top of the water. Its unfolding petals suggest the expansion of the soul. The beauty of the flower, rising from the mud of its origin, represents the divine spark of goodness within us all. The spine must be kept perfectly straight while performing the Lotus, a reminder that man is the only creature on earth with a vertical spine and, as mentioned previously, is considered to be the mystical link between heaven and earth.

The hand position utilized in the Lotus is also highly symbolic. The thumb represents God, truth, light, the infinite. The index and middle fingers are the two fingers used to demonstrate the individual will and the desire of one person to dominate another. For example, the index finger is used to emphasize the commands "You come here," "You do this," or "You listen to me." Pointing the index finger during a conversation is a strong body-language attempt to bring the listener under the domination of the speaker's words.

The joining of the thumb and index finger in a circle with the thumb on top symbolizes the bending of the individual will to the will of God. This gesture, called a *mudra*, is the equivalent of Christianity's "not my will, but thine, be done." Between sunrise and sunset the palms face upward to absorb the rays of the sun, the life-giver of the universe. Between sunset and sunrise the palms face downward, a gesture that represents conservation of the life force within.

Om—the Universal Mantra

"Om," also spelled "aum," is a mantra, a potent vibratory chant. The sound of om is uttered in order to achieve unity with God, truth, the Universal Mind.

Om means God, and it is the most ancient name for God that has been handed down through the ages. It has been used by countless millions of worshipers, always in the most universal sense; that is, referring to no one particular deity. It is symbolic of the creative force of the universe.

The word "vibrations" is a favorite of the under-thirty set, referring to that unseen but intuitively felt emanation that we all experience in regard to people, rooms, music, and just about everything else we encounter. The Om vibration, which has been called the creative hum of the Cosmic Motor, is the most powerful of all vibrations. It has three manifestations: creation, preservation, and destruction.

Words repeated over and over with deep desire and concentration gain power each time they are repeated, and have a materializing value. When Om is used in this way, man's spiritual quality increases each time it is repeated. Om is the last utterance of certain masters of India who know in advance when they are approaching their final hour on earth. These masters, in accordance with a Vedic rite, revolve the body three times, sit facing north in meditative posture, and chant "Om" as they merge with the infinite. This is called mahasamadhi.

The effect of the sound of om is calming and at the same time energizing. To experience its effectiveness, sit in a cross-legged posture, keep your spine straight, rest the hands on the knees, and form a circle with your thumb and index finger, the thumb resting on top of the index fingernail. Lower your eyelids or close eyes completely. Take a complete breath, and shape your lips to form an *O*. Slowly make the sound of *O*, using half the air in your lungs. Now close your lips, and the resulting sound will be the completion of "Om." When you have completely expelled all the air in your lungs, take another breath and repeat. Repeat at least seven times, once for each of the main spinal chakras, and concentrate fully on the sound you are making.

Individual Mantras

Om is a universal mantra; there are also individual mantras. Each person is thought to have a unique vibration in keeping with his or her role in the cosmic pattern, and also to be connected to an individual sound vibration, a divinely assigned mantra that has been that soul's own through all incarnations. The meditation process should eventually reveal to the meditator the syllables linked eternally to his or her soul. This mantra is a very personal prayer, or invocation, that is repeated during meditation to produce certain physical and psychological effects.

The mantra consists of a combination of Sanskrit phrases and also can be bestowed upon a devotee by a master teacher or guru in a ritualistic ceremony. Master teachers are those who have attained samadhi, divine union with God, and to whom all things, including the mantra assigned to each soul, are known. The bestowing of a mantra carries an obligation that the conferring master include the devotee in his daily prayers. And the mantra does not truly belong to the devotee until he or she has used it religiously for twenty-one consecutive days, when it then affords enlightenment and protection.

Although anyone seeking spiritual enlightenment can use a mantra, one branch of yoga, mantra-yoga, uses them exclusively. This branch does not utilize asanas but concentrates solely on the repetition of mantras. Enlightenment is said to take twelve years.

The Chakras

The human spine, which, as previously noted, is regarded as the mystical link between God and man, has seven centers called *chakras*, the Sanskrit word for wheels. These chakras are generators and storage centers for prana, or energy. The first chakra is located at the base of the spine and represents man's lowest nature; the uppermost chakra is located at the top of the skull and symbolizes the highest spirituality, the spark of God within all people.

In the average person most of these chakras are dormant—perhaps unfortunately, because when they are activated, the level of consciousness is raised, providing additional awareness necessary in man's search for himself.

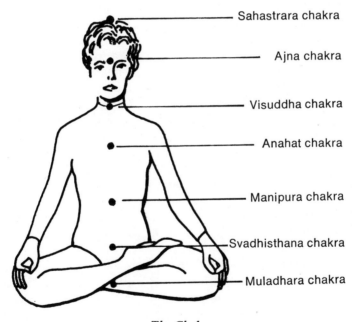

Sahastrara chakra

Ajna chakra

Visuddha chakra

Anahat chakra

Manipura chakra

Svadhisthana chakra

Muladhara chakra

The Chakras

Compare the spine and its seven chakras with a building containing seven stories. The most comprehensive view is obviously from the top floor, and the most limited range of vision occurs on the first floor. As man progresses upward, unlocking the door, or chakra, of each floor, his range of vision, or state of consciousness, expands. Depending on which chakra is involved, this expanded consciousness includes clairvoyance, telepathy, spiritual visions, knowledge of past, present, and future, and other occult faculties.

Located in the lowest vertebra in the muladhara chakra is the kundalini power, which is represented by a coiled and sleeping serpent. Once awakened, the goal of the kundalini power is to gain ascent through the spinal column, called the sushumna nadi, activate the remaining chakras, and unite with the uppermost one, the sahastrara chakra. The kundalini power is awakened through special yoga asanas and breathing exercises.

Heightened psychic ability rather than true spirituality is frequently the goal of many people who become interested in awakening the kundalini power. In spiritually advanced persons this power ascends naturally. But unless the seeker has first become completely purified physically, mentally, and spiritually, the awakening of these powers can be extremely dangerous.

Kundalini-awakening methods were shrouded in secrecy for centuries and were taught only to those whose integrity was of the highest order. These methods were then taught only by yogis and gurus whose lives were totally devoted to spiritual teachings. Western students would be well advised to concentrate on those aspects of yoga that fit our way of life and leave kundalini to those few who can handle it properly.

Each chakra contains a different number of petals that are initially pointing downward. As the kundalini ascends, the chakras spin, and the petals open, signifying the expansion of the soul and illumination. When it reaches the uppermost sahastrara chakra, total enlightenment results, and the yogi attains samadhi, union with God, the ultimate goal of all yogas.

The chakras relate to the astral body but correspond to various plexi located in the physical body. The *muladhara chakra*, located in the lowest vertebra, corresponds to the sacral plexus and controls elimination. The *svadhisthana chakra* is located opposite the genital organs and corresponds to the epigastric plexus; it controls sexual desire. The *manipura chakra* is in the navel area, corresponds to the solar plexus, and controls digestion. The fourth chakra, the *anahat chakra*, is located at heart level, corresponds to the cardiac plexus, and controls respiration. Located in the vicinity of the thyroid gland is the fifth, *vissudha chakra*, which corresponds to the pharyngeal plexus and controls speech. *Ajna chakra* is number six, located between the eyebrows, the seat of the mystical "third eye." This corresponds to the pineal gland, which Descartes thought to be the seat of the soul; this chakra controls the autonomic nervous system. The seventh chakra is *sahastrara* and is located at the top of the head and corresponds to the cortical layer of the brain.

Swamis, Yogis, and Gurus Defined

Interest in yoga has mushroomed in the West in recent years, and along with it such vocabulary additions as swami, guru, and yogi. Though they may seem to be used interchangeably, there are distinct differences in these terms.

A swami is a monk who has been initiated into the ancient Swami Order, this initiation being conducted by men who are themselves swamis. There are more than a million bona fide swamis, all of whom trace their spiritual ancestry back to Sri Shankara, who reorganized the Swami Order in the ninth century. Upon initiation, swamis exchange their given names for new ones, a part of which indicates to which of the ten subdivisions of the Swami Order they belong. They also dress in robes of ocher, or orange, the color that symbolizes renunciation. Swamis take vows of poverty, chastity, and obedience to their spiritual authority. They discard all prejudices and dedicate their lives to human brotherhood. Swami means one who seeks to achieve union with the *swa*, or self.

A swami may or may not actively participate in yoga postures, but a yogi is one who follows a definite, scientific step-by-step procedure of physical and mental discipline, the ultimate goal of which is liberation of the soul. A yogi may be married, in which case he is referred to as a yogi-householder. He remains in the world, but not of it, fulfilling earthly responsibilities as well as spiritual ones, but remaining unattached to the world's materialism.

A guru, as explained in Chapter 1, is a spiritual teacher, one who leads the student from darkness to light.

The Eight Steps of Yoga

The *Yoga Sutras* of Patanjali outline an eight-step path to self-realization which he called astanga-yoga, commonly known as raja-yoga. It is sometimes erroneously believed that Patanjali's system was concerned solely with spiritual development and that hatha yoga, the system outlined in Suatmarama's *Hatha Yoga Pradipika*, led only to physical and mental control. Actually, they are complementary systems. Spiritual development is greatly facilitated when mind and body function with complete control, discipline, and harmony. The eight limbs of astanga-yoga are:

1. Yamas—universal moral commandments
2. Niyamas—individual disciplinary observances
3. Asana—posture and body control
4. Pranayama—breath control
5. Pratyahara—control of the senses

6. Dharana—mind control and concentration
7. Dhyana—meditation
8. Samadhi—union with God and the true self

The yamas are universal rules of moral conduct for society, rules that transcend the boundaries of race, creed, color, nationality, age, and time. The five yamas are: nonviolence (*ahimsa*), nonlying (*satya*), nonstealing (*asteya*), nonwasting (*bramacharya*), and noncoveting (*aparigraha*).

The niyamas are inner qualities to be cultivated which include purity (*saucha*), contentment (*santosa*), austerity (*tapas*), self-study (*svadhyaya*), and awareness of a Higher Power (*isvara pranidhana*). The yamas and niyamas form the moral code of yoga and are a necessary prerequisite for the following stages. Without them, true spiritual development is impossible.

Nonviolence encompasses more than the biblical injunction "Thou shalt not kill" and in its highest form signifies a love of all creation. Recognizing that all the creatures of the earth are linked through the Creator, the nonviolent man refuses to cause harm to any living thing through his actions, words, or even thoughts.

Nonstealing commands that you take nothing that does not belong to you. This is far-reaching, including not only material things but also intangibles such as the plans, thoughts, or ideas of others.

Nonlying insists on complete truthfulness and honesty with others, and perhaps what is more difficult, with ourselves as well. Being honest with oneself is a true mark of maturity.

Nonwasting requires effective utilization of all our resources, including personal health, time, talent, speech, and energy as well as the material things such as food and financial means.

Noncoveting commands an understanding of the distinction between our wants and our needs. Our wants may be great, but our needs are really quite simple. Noncoveting urges that we view the possessions and accomplishments of others not with envy, greed, or frustration, but with a genuine feeling of joy and pride in our fellowman.

Purity involves the body, mind, and spirit. Physical purity is accomplished through bathing of the body, eating proper food for internal cleanliness, adequate elimination, and controlled breathing to eliminate toxins in the system. The mind must be purged of the impure emotions of anger, hatred, greed, envy, and pride. Spiritual pride, the feeling that only our approach to the Higher Power is the correct approach, must be eliminated before true spiritual purity can be achieved.

Contentment is the ability to accept one's lot in life with graciousness and to meet each circumstance without resentment or bitterness. A belief in reincarnation cultivates contentment, because each soul chooses its life path to provide opportunities for soul growth. When we understand that we elected, before birth, to meet certain trials and to learn the lessons these trials teach, the load is carried with greater ease.

Austerity is a reminder to keep our lives simple. Emerson said, "Our lives are frittered away by detail; simplify, simplify." He understood that unnecessary distractions destroy concentration and the quality of life. Simplicity is preferred in diet, dress, surroundings, and habits. Austerity prevents too great an attachment to the material things of the world, which from the yogic standpoint are unreal and illusory.

Self-study demands that we objectively look inward, viewing our thoughts, actions, goals, and progress with maturity, ever on guard against harboring feelings of self-satisfaction. Self-study teaches that life is an ongoing process, that change is inevitable, and that until death we are constantly becoming what we will be.

Awareness of a Higher Power is a reminder to always view ourselves from the proper perspective. Creative as man is, his creations are insignificant compared to those of the Creator of our universe. Observing the grandeur of our world—the changing of the seasons, the beauty of trees, mountains, rivers, stars, or a newborn baby—reminds us that the Creator is not out there, or up there, but all around us, always.

Asana (posture). The asanas are a necessary part of the yogic path, assuring a physical vehicle that is strong, sound, and free of disease. These postures with their ancient origin are designed to exercise every muscle, nerve, and gland in the body. Detractors of yoga claim that too much emphasis is placed on the physical body, but the yogi considers this body the living temple of the spirit. When the body is not functioning soundly, it creates pain and distractions that prevent the concentration necessary for the succeeding stages of yoga.

Pranayama (breath control). The easiest way to understand pranayama is to observe what happens to the breathing process when a person becomes angry. The angry person breathes in erratic fashion, but when the rage dissipates, the breathing again returns to normal. What is going on in the mind affects the breathing process. Conversely, the yogi knows that the breathing process affects the mind and learns to breathe in such a way that the mind remains calm, tranquil, and able to concentrate.

Pratyahara (control of the senses). The man who is a slave to the senses has a cruel master. An undisciplined appetite—whether in the area of food, sex, money, possessions, or power—leads to failure in life as well as in yoga. Excess amounts of food, particularly rich and unwholesome food, produce a body that is gross, unhealthy, and undisciplined. Abuse of sexual energy dissipates the life force and creates undue focus on sensuality. And a man possessed by the desire for material things is sometimes driven to immoral or unethical practices; he is also under the spell of maya, the delusion that the "things" he craves are the real elements of the world.

The phrase "You can't take it with you," referring to the money or possessions so many spend their lives seeking, is a subtle warning about the real and the unreal facets of our lives. The money or objects collected do not remain with you after what we know as death occurs; what does remain is the undying soul. Unfortunately, many of the practices employed by those driven by the senses erode the soul, retarding its spiritual growth. This will be covered more thoroughly in the chapter on reincarnation.

Controlling the senses means to withdraw all feeling and sensation from the various parts of the body until only awareness of the mind remains. Following the asanas and the complete relaxation, start with the toes and withdraw all feeling and sensation from them. Continue, disassociating yourself from your legs, lower torso, upper torso, internal organs, arms, hands, and fingers. Then mentally withdraw all feeling and sensation from your neck, scalp, face, mouth, tongue, and eyelids. Concentrate on your mind, being totally unaware of sensation in your body. At this point you may feel that your mind is greatly enlarged and all that remains of you.

Dharana (concentration or mind control). Only when the body has been stabilized through asanas, the mind steadied through breath control, and the senses mastered can concentration be accomplished. To concentrate is to hold the mind steadily on one thought, object, sound, or task. The average untrained and undisciplined mind has been compared to a chattering monkey, with random thoughts darting here and there, and even the thought on which concentration is centered is elusive. Concentration is a useful ability in all areas of life; it is absolutely essential in attaining self-knowledge, in recognizing the spark of divinity within, and in nurturing it to development. Concentration on and mental repetition of the universal mantra, Om, readies the mind for meditation, the next step.

Dhyana (meditation). When the mind holds itself steadily on one thought, object, or sound, and when this concentration is uninterrupted, the result is meditation. Meditation is covered in depth in Chapter 9. When the body, mind, senses, breath, and consciousness integrate harmoniously in meditation, illumination results—the understanding that defies description.

Samadhi (the goal of yoga). At the height of meditation the meditator passes into the state of samadhi. In samadhi the body and senses resemble those of one asleep, and yet the mind and reasoning faculties are wide awake and alert. Samadhi is a state of superconsciousness where all things are revealed, man is one with his Creator, and in deep peace and joy. Samadhi is the goal of all yogas.

Yoga Exercises

In the following pages are listed more than one hundred yoga postures and exercises, with appropriate photographs, and including precise, step-by-step instructions for proper and safe execution.

Before you start, read the entire asana section carefully. Then, if you are a beginner, work through the following Lesson Plan for Beginners. Be sure you study the instructions carefully and understand them before attempting a posture. When you can perform all of the postures in the Lesson Plan for Beginners, go on to the Basic Lesson Plan.

Plateaus

Once you have mastered the postures, you may find a "so what?" feeling creeping into your consciousness. Should this happen, you have reached a plateau. Without attention, these plateaus can lead to boredom and a general lack of enthusiasm, but if you recognize these halts in the learning process for what they are, you can turn them into stepping stones to greater achievement.

Left to our own devices, most of us take the path of least resistance. In working out of a plateau, you must overcome your ennui and push yourself beyond what you can do comfortably and with ease.

If you can maintain the Headstand easily for three minutes, force yourself to stay up three and a half minutes, and then four minutes. If you would like to abandon the Plough after one minute, tell your hamstrings to relax and maintain the posture for two minutes. Then add a variation, and hold that for two minutes.

If you have any doubt about your physical ability to perform postures or exercises, see your physician before undertaking this program.

LESSON PLAN FOR BEGINNERS

1. Lie in Corpse pose and completely relax: one or two minutes (page 185).
2. Eye and neck exercises (pages 86–87).
3. Spine Rock, Beginning (page 88).
4. Hamstring Stretches, lying down: two times (page 178).
5. Sun Salutation: four times (pages 90–94). This will seem awkward at first but eventually will become a rhythmic, flowing series of movements.
6. Half Shoulder Stand: one half minute (page 94).
7. Shoulder Stand: one half minute (page 97).
8. Plough: one half minute (page 99).
9. Fish: one half minute (page 103). Before trying the Fish, take this simple test: Lie on back, then raise upper body, supporting weight on elbows. The buttocks remain on the floor. Then drop head backward. If this position makes you dizzy, it is advisable to eliminate the Fish until the test no longer disturbs you.
10. Cobra: three times (page 105).
11. Half Locust: three times (page 108).
12. Bow: three times (page 110).
13. Leg Pulls: three times (page 122). When you are able to bring the head close to the knees in this, substitute the Head-to-Knee Post (page 125) and the Forward Bend here (page 104).
14. Full Spinal Twist: three times each side (page 111).
15. Triangle (page 129).
16. Breathing Exercises—Rhythmic Breathing (page 37).
17. Complete relaxation: ten minutes (page 185). Do not omit this.

Note: When you can work through the Lesson Plan for Beginners easily, proceed to the Basic Lesson Plan (below). Use the Basic Lesson Plan daily and add to it exercises and asanas specifically designated to correct any health or beauty problem you may have.

BASIC LESSON PLAN

1. Lie in Corpse pose and completely relax for one or two minutes (page 185).
2. Eye and neck exercises (pages 86–87).
3. Spine Rock, Beginning and Intermediate (pages 88–89).
4. Sun Salutation: six times (pages 90–94).
5. Headstand—when you have mastered it (page 116). Until then, substitute the Pose of Tranquillity (page 96), the Tripod (page 114), or the Half Headstand (page 115).
6. Cobra (page 105).
7. Half Locust (page 108).
8. Bow (page 110).
9. Head-to-Knee Post (page 125).
10. Forward Bend (page 104).
11. Half Shoulder Stand (page 94)—or Pose of Tranquillity (page 96).
12. Shoulder Stand (page 97).
13. Plough (page 99).
14. Fish (page 103).
15. Full Spinal Twist (page 111).
16. Triangle (page 129).
17. Camel (page 135).
18. Breathing exercises (page 37). Be sure to include alternate breathing.
19. Corpse (page 185). Complete relaxation for at least ten minutes. Do not omit this.

To this Basic Lesson Plan add exercises and asanas specifically designated to correct any health or beauty problems you may have.

EYE EXERCISES

PRECAUTION: The eye exercises outlined below should not be done while wearing contact lenses

DIRECTIONS: Step 1: Sit or stand with spine straight, shoulders back, and chin parallel to the floor, with eyes looking straight ahead. Without moving the head, look diagonally up and to the right as far as you can. Then look diagonally down and to the left. Repeat three times. Then reverse this, looking diagonally up to the left and down to the right, three times.

Step 2: Without moving the head, look straight up toward the ceiling, then down toward the floor. Repeat three times.

Step 3: Still without moving the head, look as far to the right as you can, then as far to the left as possible. Repeat three times.

Step 4: Now move the eyes in a wide circular movement to the right as though you were following an object being moved in a circular pattern. Repeat three times. Then reverse the movement, circling three times to the left.

Step 5: Now extend the left arm straight out in front of you and point the index finger toward the ceiling, with the end of that finger at eye level. Point the right index finger toward the ceiling at a spot approximately half the distance between the left index finger and your eyes. Focus both eyes first on the farther left index finger, then focus both eyes on the closer right index finger. Repeat three times.

NECK EXERCISES

DIRECTIONS: Step 1: Sit in Lotus, Half Lotus, or Easy Pose, thumb and forefinger forming a circle, with the thumb on top. Rest the hands on the knees, palms up between sunrise and sunset, down between sunset and sunrise. Keep your spine straight, with shoulders back and chin parallel to the floor, eyes looking straight ahead. Without moving your shoulders, turn your head as far as you can to the right, trying to look at the wall behind you. Then turn your head as far as you can to the left, making sure the shoulders do not move. Repeat four times in each direction.

Step 2: Still with motionless shoulders, drop your head forward toward your chest, then back until you are looking at the ceiling. It is normal for the mouth to be open as you look toward the ceiling. Repeat forward and backward movements four times.

Step 3: With eyes looking straight ahead, drop your head sideways, as though you were trying to touch your right shoulder with your right ear. Make sure the movement is directly to the side and that the shoulders do not rise as you drop your head. Then make the same movement to the left. Repeat four times on each side.

Step 4: Let your head drop forward toward your chest. Then, in one *slow* continuous movement, roll head around toward the right shoulder, then to the back, to the left shoulder, and back to the front. Continue the movement without pausing until four complete neck rolls have been performed rotating toward the right. Then reverse the movement and perform four neck rolls toward the left. The shoulders should remain motionless throughout the entire exercise.

SPINE ROCK
(Beginning)

BENEFITS: Basic warm-up • Corrects minor spinal misalignments • Eases tension in back and shoulders • Helps eliminate insomnia

PRECAUTIONS: Use adequately padded surface under spine • Avoid garments with back zipper • Tuck the chin so you will not rock on the upper spinal (cervical) vertebrae, which tend to calcify with age and lack of use

DIRECTIONS: Sit on a thick mat or well-padded floor. Bend the knees so you can place your hands just above the backs of the knees as shown. Tuck your chin into your upper chest, curve the back, and rock gently back and forth on your spine. Come back up to a sitting position at the end of each spine rock. The rocking back and up should be a continual, rhythmic movement. Continue until the spine feels loose and relaxed. After this becomes comfortable and easy, and you have done it for several weeks, try the Intermediate Spine Rock.

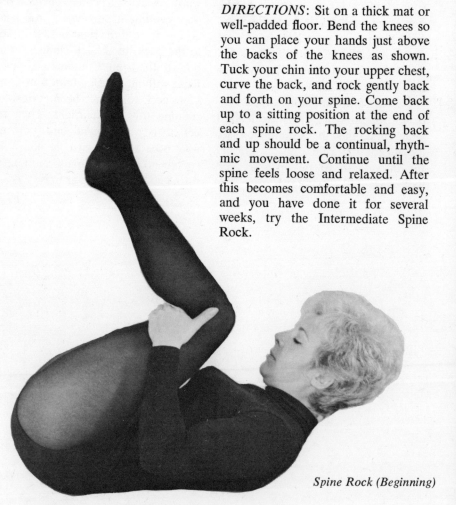

Spine Rock (Beginning)

SPINE ROCK
(Intermediate)

DIRECTIONS: Sit with bent knees close to torso, cross the ankles, and grasp left toes in right hand and right toes in left hand. Rock back on the spine as before, and still holding the toes, extend the legs so toes touch the floor. After rocking up to a sitting position, bend down from the lowest part of your spine so that you can touch the floor in front of your feet with your forehead while keeping the buttocks on the mat.

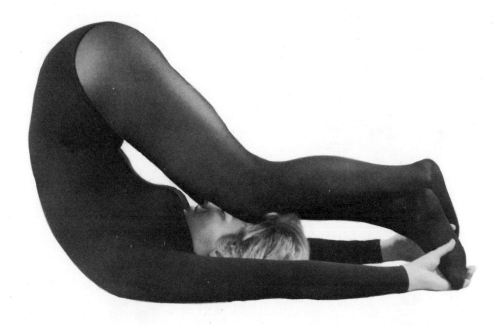

Spine Rock (Intermediate)

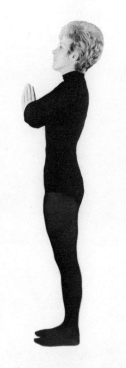

Sun Salutation—Step 1

SUN SALUTATION

Traditionally, the Sun Salutation is performed twelve times at dawn, facing east, while addressing the Lord of the Sun by his twelve different names. For beginners, two to six times through the sequence is a good introduction. This should be done daily.

BENEFITS: All-purpose warm-up for stretching all the muscles and ligaments of the body

PRECAUTIONS: If you have a weak or damaged back, be extremely careful while doing Steps 2 and 11. In these steps bend the knees more so there is not an extreme arch in the spine.

DIRECTIONS: Step 1: Stand erect with feet an inch or so apart for balance, and fold the hands in front of the chest.

Step 2: Inhale, and bend backward with arms raised. Allow your knees to bend slightly, and try to look at the wall behind you.

Step 3: Exhale as you bend forward, trying to touch your toes, or ideally to place your palms on the

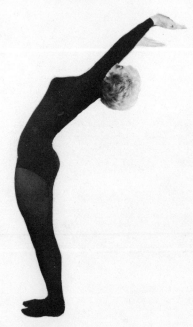

Sun Salutation—Step 2

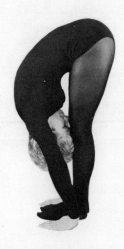

Sun Salutation—Step 3

floor. The hands remain on the floor without moving through Step 10. Keep your knees as straight as possible, and try to touch your head to your knees.

Step 4: Inhale, and stretch the left leg out behind you, placing that knee on the floor. The right foot is between your hands, which are flat on the floor. Stretch your neck to look at the ceiling.

Step 5: Retain breath, straighten left knee, and extend right leg back beside the left leg. Your body should be in a straight line with the weight resting on hands and toes. Focus your eyes on a spot on the floor eighteen inches ahead of your hands.

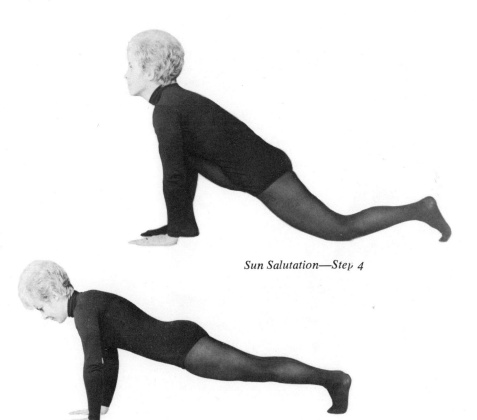

Sun Salutation—Step 4

Sun Salutation—Step 5

Step 6: Exhale as you drop your knees to the floor, then your forehead, and finally your chest. Your back is arched, keeping the abdomen off the floor. Eight points of your body touch the floor: both feet, both knees, both hands, forehead, and chest. In preparation for the next position unflex the ankles so the backs of the feet are on the floor with toes pointing out behind you. Keep your hands in position, and lower the abdomen so the front of the body is flat on the floor.

Step 7: Inhale, and slowly raise the head and upper body bending backward as far as possible.

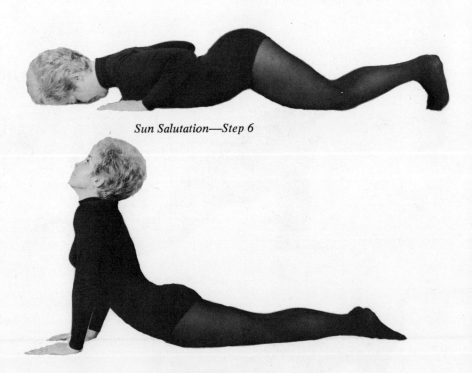

Sun Salutation—Step 6

Sun Salutation—Step 7

Step 8: Exhale as you flex the ankles, reversing the position of the toes. Lift the body, keeping the knees straight, and try to press the heels down on the floor. The body position forms a triangle.

Step 9: Inhale, and bring the left leg up between your hands. If you can't get into this position with one giant step, use your toes in inchworm fashion to inch your foot into position. This is the same as Step 4, with the right knee on the floor and the neck stretched to look at the ceiling.

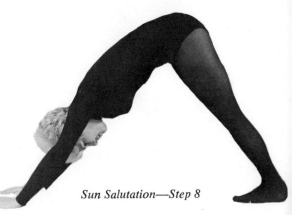

Sun Salutation—Step 8

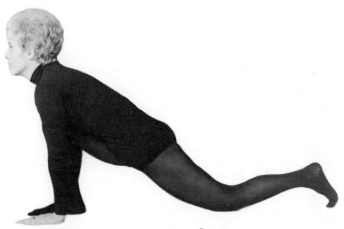

Sun Salutation—Step 9

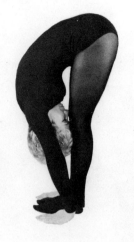

Sun Salutation—Step 10

Step 10: Exhale, and repeat Step 3 with hands touching toes, knees straight, and head trying to touch the knees.

Step 11: Inhale, bringing the hands up and bending backward as in Step 2.

Step 12: Exhale, and bring palms together in front of chest as in Step 1.

HALF SHOULDER STAND

BENEFITS: Prevents and eliminates wrinkles • Firms facial tissue • Stimulates glands and nervous centers in the brain • Good inverted posture for those who have not mastered the Headstand

PRECAUTIONS: Do not attempt if your blood pressure is lower than 100 or higher than 150, or if you have weak eye capillaries. This also applies to the Pose of Tranquillity.

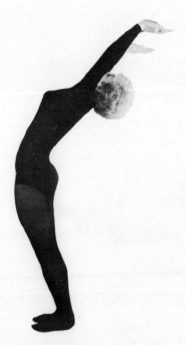

Sun Salutation—Step 11

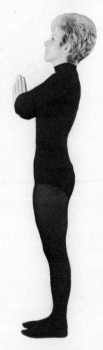

Sun Salutation—Step 12

DIRECTIONS: Lie flat on your back with arms at sides, palms down. Relax completely for a moment, then inhale, and *slowly* raise the straightened legs until they are at right angles to the body. Pause a moment to exhale, then on inhalation continue raising the body until the buttocks leave the floor and the legs are at a 45° angle to the floor, the hands supporting the hips as shown. Breathe deeply and rhythmically, and hold the posture for thirty seconds to start, adding a few seconds each day. This posture is a good preliminary for the full Shoulder Stand which follows on the next page, and you can go directly into the Shoulder Stand from the Half Shoulder Stand. As you become more proficient, you can substitute the Pose of Tranquillity for the Half Shoulder Stand.

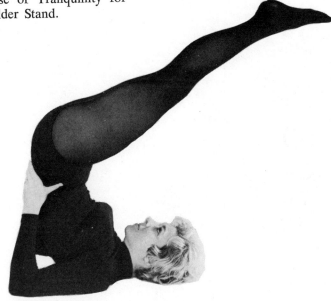

Half Shoulder Stand

POSE OF TRANQUILLITY

BENEFITS: Same as for the Half Shoulder Stand, plus being a very effective natural tranquilizer that improves balance

DIRECTIONS: Assume the Half Shoulder Stand, then place the hands on the fronts of the legs as shown. The legs must be at a 45° angle to the floor, and the arms are held straight. Where the hands are placed

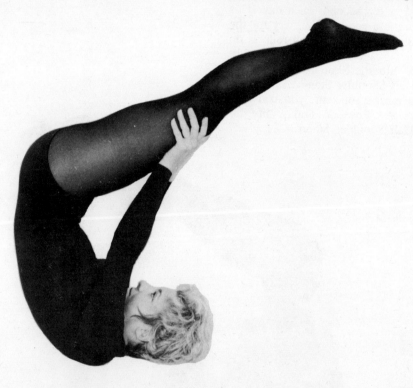

Pose of Tranquillity

on the legs will be determined by your individual proportions. Let the weight of your legs rest on your arms, which sets your balance. Hold this posture for thirty seconds to start, and gradually add a few seconds each day until you can hold the posture for five minutes. Both the Half Shoulder Stand and the Pose of Tranquillity are completed in the same manner as the full Shoulder Stand, which is shown.

SHOULDER STAND

BENEFITS: Weight regulator for both overweight and underweight due to stimulation of the thyroid gland • Eliminates constipation • All-purpose energizer • Circulation stimulator • Super-stretcher for muscles and ligaments in the cervical region of the spine • Strengthens the entire spine • Aids sinus problems • Helps reduce varicose veins

PRECAUTIONS: Do not attempt the Shoulder Stand if your blood pressure is lower than 100 or higher than 150, or if you have weak eye capillaries • Do not press the chin tightly into the chest if you have a hyperactive thyroid gland • Approach this position cautiously if you have had a whiplash or similar neck injury • Do not attempt to turn your head while in this position

DIRECTIONS: Lie flat on your back with arms at sides, palms down. Relax completely for a moment, then inhale, and slowly raise the straightened legs until they are at right angles to the body. Pause a moment to ex-

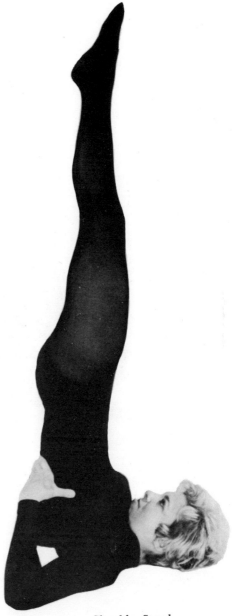

Shoulder Stand

hale, then on inhalation continue raising the body until the buttocks and back leave the floor and the hands are positioned on the back for support as shown. Your weight is resting on the neck and shoulders, and your chin must be pressing firmly into the base of the neck. Breathe deeply and rhythmically, and hold the posture for thirty seconds to start, working up gradually to as long as fifteen minutes. Try to keep the body straight. Don't just collapse out of this posture! Place both hands flat on the floor as shown below, lower the knees to the forehead, and finally lower your trunk to the floor. Then straighten your knees, and *slowly* lower your legs to the floor.

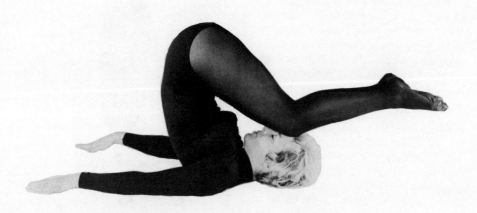

Shoulder Stand (Completion)

SHOULDER BALANCE
(Variation of the Shoulder Stand)

BENEFITS: Same as for Shoulder Stand, plus improved balance

PRECAUTIONS: Same as for Shoulder Stand

DIRECTIONS: Assume the full Shoulder Stand. To assume this balance posture, slowly move your arms alongside the outer thighs, being careful to maintain balance. Try to hold this for one minute, gradually increasing the time up to three minutes. The Shoulder Balance is completed in the same manner as the full Shoulder Stand.

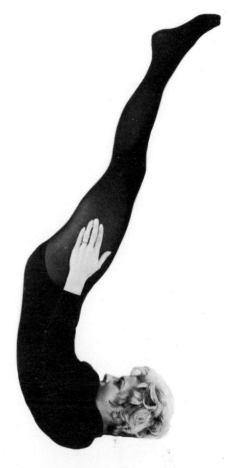

Shoulder Balance

PLOUGH

BENEFITS: Spinal flexibility • Reduces the abdomen and hips • Stretches the hamstrings • Strengthens the neck • Rejuvenates sex glands, liver, kidneys, and spleen • Regulates weight through stimulation of the thyroid

PRECAUTIONS: If you have a hyperactive thyroid gland, avoid pressing the chin into the chest too tightly • Proceed with caution if you have had a whiplash or similar neck injury • Do not allow your legs to drop or fall into this position quickly; bring them down *in control* while supporting your hips to prevent sudden undue pressure on the neck

DIRECTIONS: Assume the full Shoulder Stand position. Inhale, and *slowly* lower the legs to the floor over your head as you exhale. Be sure to support the body with the hands as the legs are being lowered. If you cannot touch the floor, go as far as you can; each time you attempt the posture, your toes will come closer to the floor. If you find your legs are shaky on the descent, press the feet and legs together firmly. Place your arms over your head as shown. At first, hold the posture motionless for thirty seconds, and repeat it three times. As you become more proficient, perform it once, and hold for two minutes. As you become more flexible, curve the toes back toward the body, working eventually toward getting the feet flat on the floor.

In Variation #1 the hands are placed flat on the floor. (This variation does not greatly stimulate the thyroid and is of less value as a weight regulator.) Beginners will notice that the wrists tend to raise off the floor as shown. When the posture

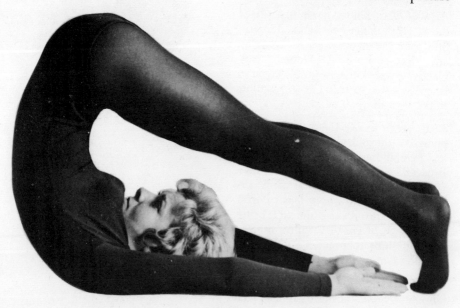

Plough

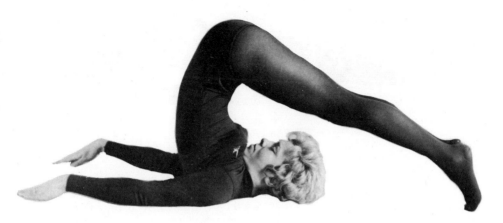

Plough—Variation #1

becomes easier, work toward keeping the wrists down and the arms parallel to each other. This posture is completed in the same manner as the Shoulder Stand.

FISH
(Beginning)

BENEFITS: The Fish normally follows the Plough (page 99) in order to reverse the spinal curve, and beneficially affects the entire spine • Increases circulation to cervical spine and shoulder area and removes stiffness from these areas • Improves asthmatic conditions

PRECAUTIONS: Proceed cautiously if you have had a whiplash or similar neck injury • If the posture makes you dizzy, it indicates that the carotid arteries supplying blood to the brain are being compressed too greatly. Reposition the head so there is a less acute angle and less pressure on the

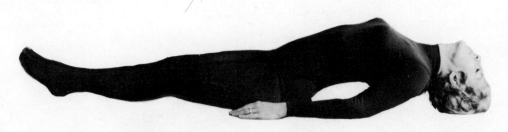

Fish (Beginning)

neck. Inner ear irregularities also cause dizziness, and the Fish is prohibited when this condition exists.

DIRECTIONS: Lie flat on back with arms relaxed at your sides. With palms flat on the floor, inhale, and raise chest using elbows for support. Bend your neck backward, arching back sharply, and place the top of your head on the floor. *The buttocks are not raised off the floor.* Now remove pressure from the elbows so that the arms lie relaxed beside your body and your weight is supported by the top of your head and buttocks. Breathe deeply and rhythmically. Hold for thirty seconds to start, working up gradually to two minutes. To come out of the Fish, place elbows on floor for support, lift head, and slowly lower the back until again lying flat.

Note: After you have practiced yoga for several weeks, a good sequence is to perform two minutes each of the Half Shoulder Stand, Shoulder Stand, Plough, and Fish and then "float," which means to lie flat on your back, completely relaxed, for two minutes.

FISH WITH CROSSED ANKLES
(Intermediate)

BENEFITS: Provides counteracting spinal stretch following Shoulder Stand • Stimulates thyroid • Removes stiffness from cervical spine • Helps reduce spasms in the bronchial area, which plague asthmatics

PRECAUTIONS: Do not arch the neck too sharply if you have a hyperactive thyroid

DIRECTIONS: Sit in tailor fashion with both knees bent and the ankles crossed. Lean back on the elbows, then arch the back sharply, and place the top of the head on the floor. The weight is borne by the head and the buttocks. Now reach down, and grasp the right toes with the left hand and the left toes with the right hand. Try to bring the knees down to the floor. Hold for thirty seconds at first, working up to two minutes.

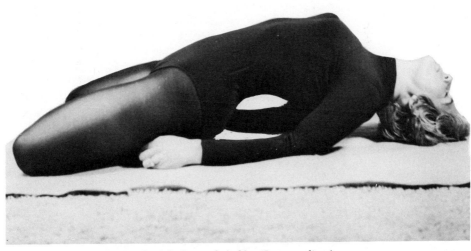

Fish with Crossed Ankles (Intermediate)

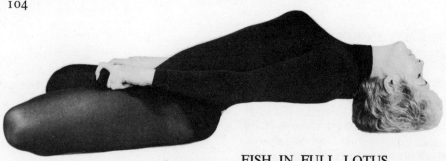

Fish in Full Lotus (Advanced)

FISH IN FULL LOTUS
(Advanced)

DIRECTIONS: Sit in Full Lotus, lean back on the elbows, then arch the back sharply, and place the top of the head on the floor. Then grasp the big toes with the index fingers as shown. Hold for thirty seconds at first, working up to two minutes.

FORWARD BEND
(Posterior Stretch or Stretching Posture)

BENEFITS: Removes fat from the abdomen and hips • Strengthens abdominal muscles • Tones up the nervous system • Increases flexibility in the lumbar region of the spine • Stretches the hamstrings • Gently massages all the abdominal organs • Restores sexual vigor • Eliminates constipation and aids digestion • Helps control diabetes through stimulation of the pancreas

PRECAUTIONS: None

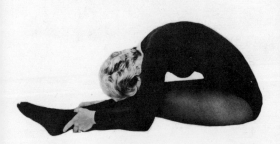

Forward Bend

DIRECTIONS: Lie flat on your back with straightened arms placed on the floor over your head. Interlock your thumbs, and raise the arms until fingers are pointing toward the ceiling. Without pausing, lift the head *but not the shoulders*, and continue the movement of the arms until the hands come to rest on the fronts of the thighs. Now curve the back, and slowly, vertebra by vertebra, lift the back from the mat. Still keeping the back curved, slide the hands forward toward the toes. Grasp the ankles, and hold the posture motionless for a count of ten; repeat three times. When you first practice this posture, unless your spine is unusually flexible, there will be space between the legs and chest as shown. As your spine and hamstrings loosen, work toward placing your chest directly on top of your legs without space between them. When you can do this, hook the index fingers around the big toe, and gradually lengthen the time you remain in this posture until you can hold it from two to five minutes.

COBRA

Although the Cobra, Half Locust, and Bow are separate exercises, they are most effectively used in sequence to totally flex, limber, and loosen the spine.

BENEFITS: Removes tension from spine • Improves digestion • Stimulates liver, gallbladder, pancreas, and

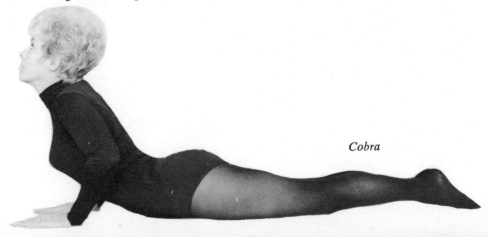

Cobra

spleen • Combats constipation • Improves some forms of sciatica • Improves posture • Builds up chest and bust • Firms chin and jawline • Beneficially affects the entire nervous system

PRECAUTIONS: Those who have a hyperactive thyroid should not bend the neck back so sharply that undue pressure is exerted on the front of the neck

DIRECTIONS: Lie on stomach with palms on floor, the ends of the fingers being in line with the top of the shoulder. Relax completely, then on inhalation brush the floor with the forehead, nose, and chin, and slowly raise the upper body one vertebra at a time. Do not push up with your hands, but let your spine do the lifting as much as possible. When you have raised as high as you can using the spine and back muscles, push with your hands to bend the body backward as far as you can (*page 105*) *while keeping the navel on the floor*. Breathe normally, and hold for a count of ten. On exhalation begin lowering the body from the lowest part of the spine, vertebra by vertebra, letting the spine do the lowering. Keep your eyes on the ceiling as you lower; and to complete the posture, brush the floor with the chin, nose, and finally the forehead. Take a complete breath, and relax all the muscles in the body. Repeat three times.

COBRA—
Variation #1

BENEFITS: Improves the bustline • Strengthens the arms and spine • Im-

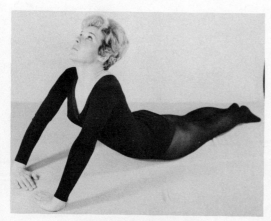

Cobra—Variation #1

parts awareness of each individual vertebra • Firms under-chin area

PRECAUTIONS: Be extremely careful if you have a bad back

DIRECTIONS: Lie on stomach with hands at shoulder level, palms down, fingers pointing toward each other. Inhale, and slowly push the upper body off the mat until the arms are straight and you are looking toward the ceiling; hold for a count of ten. Keeping eyes upward, begin exhaling, and slowly start pressing the front of your body against the mat. The arms provide a bit of resistance, and you will feel that there is not quite enough space for your body, that your spine is being compressed somewhat. Repeat three times. This variation is quite different from the classic Cobra, in which the elbows are bent, the spine is used to lift the upper body, and the navel remains on the floor.

COBRA—
Variation #2

BENEFITS: Same as the classic Cobra, plus increased flexibility and range of movement for the neck

PRECAUTIONS: Be careful if you have had a whiplash or similar neck injury

DIRECTIONS: Perform the Cobra according to the directions above. When the upper body is completely off the mat, slowly turn your head as far to the left as it will go, attempting to see your heels. Then turn your head as far as it will go to the right,

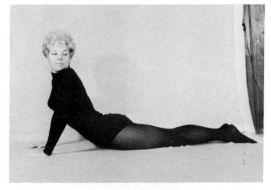

Cobra—Variation #2

return to center position, stretch your neck to look at the ceiling, and slowly lower your body to the mat while keeping your eyes upturned.

HALF LOCUST

BENEFITS: Strengthens back muscles • Provides an internal massage for the kidneys which improves diuretic action • Firms and trims the buttocks·and thighs • Revitalizes the nervous system • Improves low-back pain when discomfort is due to weak muscles • Prevents or improves varicose veins through improved blood circulation in the legs • Normalizes intestinal action and prevents constipation

PRECAUTIONS: None

DIRECTIONS: Relax completely for a moment while lying flat on your

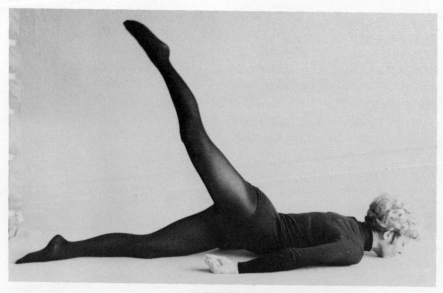

Half Locust

stomach with the chin pushed forward on floor or mat. Your legs should be straight, feet together, and toes pointed. The arms are straight and close to the body. Clench your fists, and place the backs of your hands against the floor. Inhale, and raise the right leg as high as you can *without rolling over to the left or bending the knee*. The leg can be raised much higher if you do roll to the left, but this minimizes the effects of the posture and is to be avoided. Hold for a count of five, and lower the leg back to the floor on exhalation. Perform with the left leg; repeat three times.

FULL LOCUST

The Full Locust is an advanced variation of the Half Locust and is far more difficult to perform. In attempting this posture, don't be discouraged if your feet can be raised only a few inches off the floor. The fully executed posture shown here requires extreme flexibility in the lumbar region of the spine and great muscular strength. It is a much easier posture for men than for women.

DIRECTIONS: In this posture the hands are interlocked and placed under the body. In one powerful thrusting motion, raise the legs, trying to get them as nearly vertical as possible.

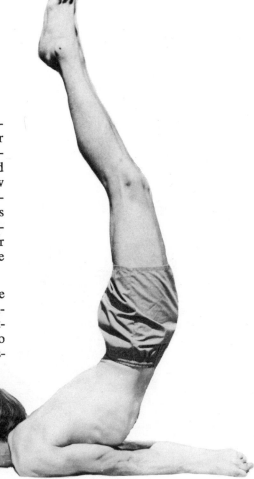

Full Locust

BOW

BENEFITS: Reinforces benefits of both the Cobra and the Locust • Improves posture • Eases tension in back and shoulders • Benefits circulation and digestion • Develops the chest and bust • Strengthens muscles of back and abdomen

PRECAUTIONS: Approach this cautiously if you have a back problem

DIRECTIONS: Lie on floor or mat, face down, and relax completely for a moment. Bend the knees, and reach back to take a firm grasp of the ankles. Inhale, and raise the knees and head simultaneously as though the body were a bow and the arms a bowstring. Push your feet firmly against your hands to lift the head and knees as high as possible. Hold for a count of five, then exhale, and slowly lower head and knees to floor.

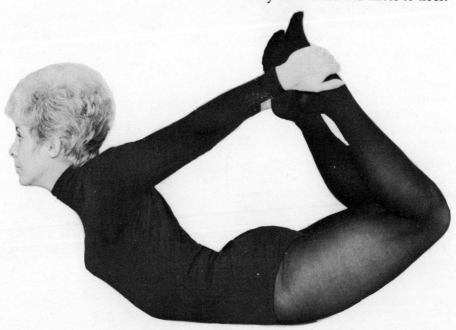

Bow

Relax. Repeat three times. It may be difficult at first to raise head and knees very far off the floor. Be sure to push away from your hands with your feet, as this is how the body is raised. Advanced students may rock back and forth on the abdomen, inhaling as the body rocks backward and exhaling as the head rocks toward the floor.

FULL SPINAL TWIST

BENEFITS: Increases spinal flexibility • Twisting to the right stimulates the liver and right kidney • Twisting to the left stimulates the pancreas, spleen, and left kidney • Eliminates constipation • Aids the nervous system

PRECAUTIONS: Be sure to compress the right side of the abdomen first in order to work in conjunction with the normal peristaltic action of the intestines. To compress the right side of the abdomen, initiate the posture by first bending the left knee; to compress the left side, begin by bending the right knee.

DIRECTIONS: From a sitting position, bend the left knee, and bring heel to position shown. Place right foot flat on floor at left of bent left knee. The left knee and the right heel should be on the same level. Bring left arm alongside outer side of upraised right knee, and grasp instep of right foot. If you cannot reach the instep, try to grasp the right ankle or the left knee. With the lower body firmly anchored, begin twisting to the right from the lowermost spine. Now twist your right arm and shoulder and

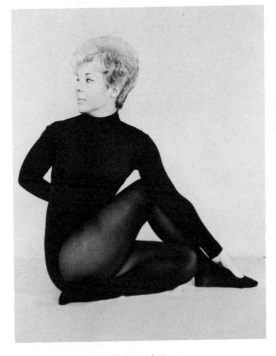

Full Spinal Twist

finally your head as far as possible to the right. Stretch your right arm behind you, placing palm down on your back at waist level. As you become more flexible, you may be able to grasp the right knee with the right hand. Keep your trunk balanced and upright. Breathe deeply and rhythmically, and hold the posture from three to ten complete breaths. Reverse directions, and twist to the opposite side. You will notice that twisting will be easier on one side.

Lotus

LOTUS

Here is a simple test to see if your thigh joints are ready to attempt the Lotus. Sit on the floor with legs outstretched. Bend the right knee, and place the sole of the foot against the left inner thigh as high up as possible. Now push the right knee with a bouncing motion trying to make it touch the floor. Reverse legs, and try to get the other knee down to the floor. You may be able to do it the first time, but it may take days, weeks, or months to be able to bounce the knees down to the floor.

BENEFITS: Stretches thigh, knee, and ankle joints • Provides a firm seat for meditation

PRECAUTIONS: Do not attempt the Lotus until you can pass the above test • Do not hold for longer than thirty seconds if you have varicose veins

DIRECTIONS: Sit with legs outstretched, bend right knee, take right foot in both hands and place it, sole

upward, on top of left thigh. Now
bend left knee, grasp left foot, and
try to glide it on top of right thigh.
Try to maintain this posture for thirty
seconds, increasing it by ten seconds
daily until it is comfortable for as
long as five minutes.

YOGA MUDRA

BENEFITS: Stretches the spine and
makes it more flexible • This is the
posture that is said to be a specific
for those with excess pride

PRECAUTIONS: Do not hold this
posture for more than thirty seconds
if you have varicose veins

DIRECTIONS: Assume the Lotus
posture. If you have not yet mastered
the Lotus, sit cross-legged in the Easy
Pose or in the Half Lotus (*page 166*).
Imagine a hook attached to the top of
your head pulling you up taller and

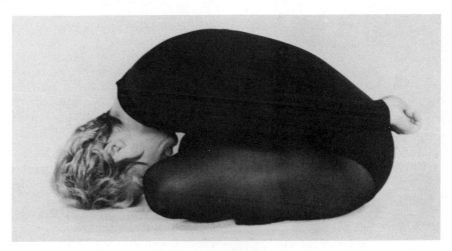

Yoga Mudra

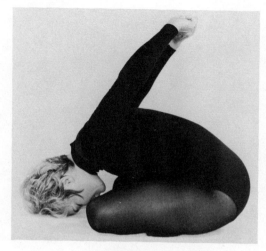

Yoga Mudra—Variation

taller. Now bend forward, beginning at the lowermost vertebra. Continue bending forward slowly, vertebra by vertebra, feeling the stretching movement throughout the spine. It may help to keep the face forward until the very last moment when you place the forehead on the floor. Place hands behind you, the right wrist lightly grasping the left as shown; hold for as long as possible, breathing deeply.

Variation: In the variation the straightened arms are raised as high as possible; this variation also corrects round shoulders and improves posture.

TRIPOD

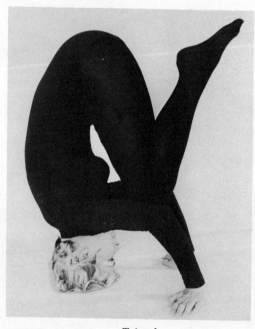

Tripod

BENEFITS: Accustoms students to being upside down in preparation for the Headstand • Combats aging by reversing the pull of gravity • Increases circulation in face and head, which improves the complexion and lessens wrinkles

PRECAUTIONS: All inverted postures are prohibited for those with blood pressure over 150 or under 100 and for those with hardening of the arteries • Avoid this if you have weak eye capillaries, glaucoma, or other eye disorders such as a detached retina • Do not perform while you have an ear infection

DIRECTIONS: Assume a position on the floor on hands and knees with fingers pointing out to the sides as shown. Stretch your head and neck forward as far as is comfortable, and place crown of head on the floor. Now straighten the knees so that legs and back form a pyramid shape. Your elbows should be no more than twelve to fourteen inches apart. Slowly walk forward on the toes until you can place knees on elbows and remain balanced there. Hold for thirty seconds, and repeat three times, relaxing between repetitions. Gradually add more time until you can hold for two minutes.

HALF HEADSTAND
(Pyramid Posture)

BENEFITS: Prepares beginning students for the Headstand and replaces the Headstand for those with unsound necks and those psychologically unsuited to the completed posture • Improves circulation and complexion • Retards the aging process by reversing the pull of gravity • Replaces the Tripod for those with a disproportionately long femur (thighbone) who cannot balance in that posture

PRECAUTIONS: Prohibited for those with high or low blood pressure, weak eye capillaries, glaucoma, or the threat of a detached retina

DIRECTIONS: Kneeling, place elbows on floor or mat. The distance between elbows equals the length of the forearm. Without moving the elbows, lightly interlock fingers. Straighten the knees so the body resembles a pyramid. At this time, consciously think "down with the elbows." Slowly walk forward, keeping knees straight, as far as you can go without bending knees. Hold for a

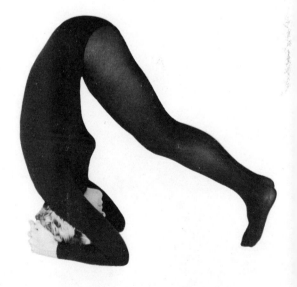

Half Headstand (Pyramid Posture)

count of ten; repeat three times. Gradually increase the time this is held up to two minutes; at that point perform the Half Headstand only once.

HEADSTAND

BENEFITS: Produces body symmetry • Slims the hips and builds up the chest • Aids memory and complexion by increasing flow of blood to the head • Repositions sagging abdominal organs • Aids varicose veins • Tones up the endocrine system • Generally benefits the entire organism

PRECAUTIONS: Prohibited for those with blood pressure over 150 or under 100, heart disorders, or hardening of the arteries • Do not attempt if you have weak eye capillaries, glaucoma, or have been warned of the possibility of a detached retina • Proceed cautiously if you have had a neck injury

DIRECTIONS: The key to performing the Headstand, I think, is to learn to think "down with the elbows" rather than "up with the feet." The Headstand is done step by step. Be sure you can do each step with ease and assurance before going to the next.

Step 1: Kneeling, place elbows on carpeted floor, mat, or folded blanket. The distance between elbows

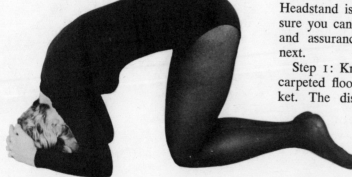

Headstand—Step 1

equals the length of your forearm. Without moving the elbows, lightly interlock the fingers on the floor, cradling the head against interlocked fingers.

Step 2: Straighten the knees so the body resembles a pyramid. At this time, consciously think "down with the elbows."

Step 3: Slowly walk forward keeping knees straight until fronts of thighs are close to chest. Keep thinking "down with the elbows."

Step 4: Slowly, in control, lift feet off floor, still thinking "down with the elbows" and maintaining balance.

Step 5: Slowly raise legs, keeping thighs close to chest. Keep raising until the legs are upright. Continued concentration on the elbows keeps the body from flipping over.

Step 6: To come down, bend knees and thigh joints, and slowly return to the starting position. Lie down for at least one minute after completing the Headstand. Try to hold the Headstand for thirty seconds at first, and work up to three minutes.

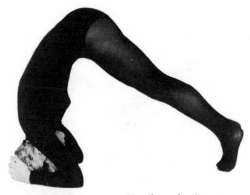

Headstand—Step 2

Headstand—Step 3

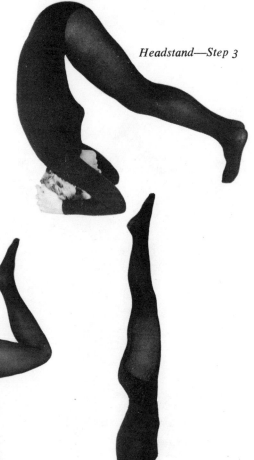

Headstand—Step 4

Headstand—Step 5

Headstand—Completed Posture

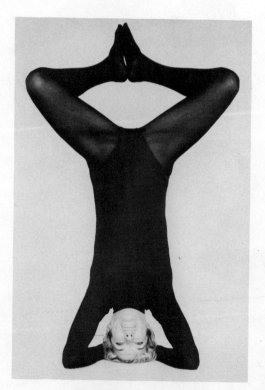

Headstand—Variation #1

HEADSTAND VARIATIONS

Once the Headstand has been mastered, there are variations that make holding the posture more interesting. Each variation has its own benefits, as well as those of the Headstand.

Variation #1: In the Headstand spread the legs as far apart as possible, which firms the inner thighs.

Variation #2: Place the soles of the feet together as shown, which stretches the thigh joints.

Variation #3: Twist the body to the right and to the left, slowly and in control, which improves balance and increases spinal flexibility.

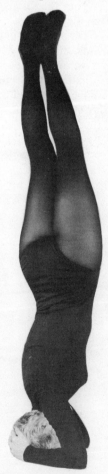

Headstand—Variation #2

Headstand, Twisting—Variation #3

Variation #4: While in the Head-stand, bring one leg down until it is parallel to the floor while the other remains upright, then reverse the legs, and continue alternating legs. As your balance improves, begin moving the upright leg farther back as the other goes frontward. Gradually increase the speed with which you perform these movements until you can scissor the legs back and forth quite rapidly.

Variation #5: While in the Head-stand, bring both straightened legs down toward the floor while keeping the trunk upright. This demands extra strength and balance and is quite demanding. When you have progressed to the point of bringing both legs down to the floor and can then lift them back up into Headstand position, try assuming the Headstand with straight legs. In other words, follow the instructions for the Headstand on page 116 through Step 3, then lift the legs into the completed posture without bending the knees. This is very difficult, so make sure your back is strong enough before you try it.

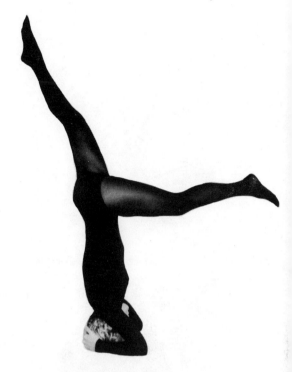

Headstand—Variation #4

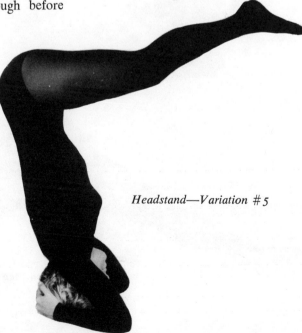

Headstand—Variation #5

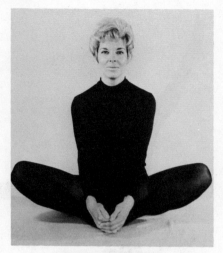

Sitting Five-Step—Step 1

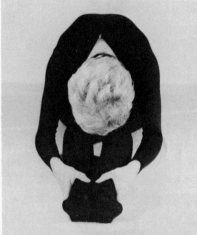

Sitting Five-Step—Step 2

SITTING FIVE-STEP

BENEFITS: Slims and firms the legs • Stretches the hamstrings • Provides flexibility for the lower back • Reduces the waistline

PRECAUTIONS: Do not force the head lower than it can go comfortably. Using undue force can injure leg muscles.

DIRECTIONS: Most yoga exercises require the holding of a posture for a specified length of time. The Sitting Five-Step is unusual, as it employs quick, repetitive movements.

Step 1: Sit on floor or mat, and place soles of feet together as shown. Then grasp toes, and bounce down, trying to bring the head as close as possible to the toes. Bounce down a total of sixteen times.

Step 2: Sit up with spine straight, extend legs straight out in front, grasp ankles lightly. Bounce down to a count of sixteen, trying to touch forehead to knees.

Sitting Five-Step—Step 3

Step 3: Sit up with spine straight, and spread the legs as far apart as is comfortable. Grasp the left ankle, and bounce down sixteen times, trying to touch forehead to left knee. Caution: Don't strain, and don't go beyond the point of pain.

Step 4: Repeat Step 3 on the right side.

Step 5: Sit up straight, and with outstretched arms, bounce down sixteen times between spread legs, trying to touch forehead to the floor. Repeat each of the five steps, bouncing down to a count of eight, then four, two, and one. As you become more advanced, keep the toes pointed toward the ceiling for a more pronounced stretch of the hamstrings.

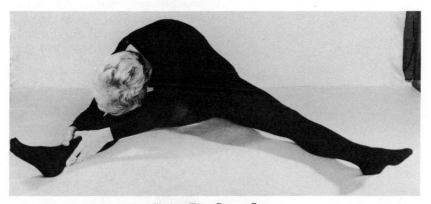

Sitting Five-Step—Step 4

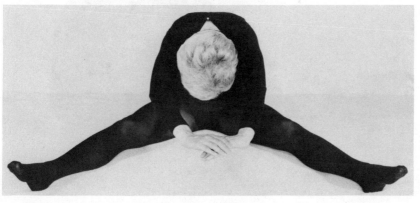

Sitting Five-Step—Step 5

LEG PULLS

BENEFITS: Replaces the Forward Bend and Head-to-Knee Post for those with very stiff lower spines or extremely tight hamstrings • Removes tension from the legs

PRECAUTIONS: Do not go beyond the point of pain

DIRECTIONS: Assume a sitting position on floor or mat with legs outstretched in front of you, feet together. Extend your arms to the front, palms down, with the backs of your hands at shoulder level. Inhale, and very slowly, bending from the lowest point of the spine, on exhalation stretch forward as far as you can without straining, placing your hands as far down on your legs as possible (*below*). This point will vary according to your spinal flexibility and may

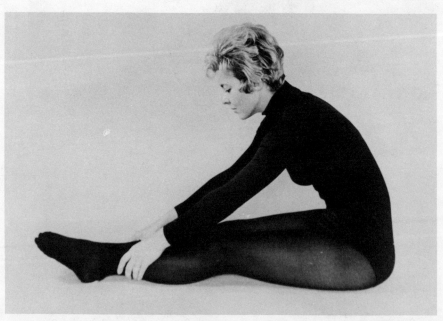

Leg Pulls

be the knee, calf, ankle, or toe. Bend your elbows, and gently pull yourself forward and downward until you are at the point beyond which you cannot go without straining. Do not push yourself beyond the point you can reach with comfort. Hold this position absolutely motionless for a count of ten. Concentrate on relaxing while in the position—don't fight it. Repeat three times; gradually increase the time the posture is held up to two minutes, and perform it only once.

WARM-UP FOR FORWARD-BENDING POSTURES

BENEFITS: Loosens the back and hamstrings in preparation for Forward Bend, the Head-to-Knee Post, and Standing Forward Bend

PRECAUTIONS: Take it easy if you have a back problem • Don't force the body in this warm-up

DIRECTIONS: Sit on floor or mat with legs stretched out in front of the

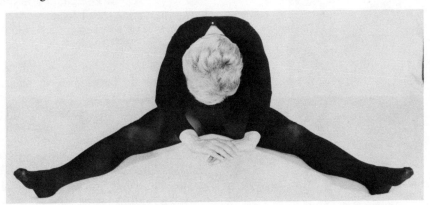

Warm-up for Forward Bending Postures

body and spread as far apart as possible, arms outstretched in front as shown. Bending from the base of the spine—not the waistline—bring the head as close as possible to the outstretched right leg. Inhale, and on exhalation make gentle, wavelike, bouncing motions as you direct the upper body toward the left leg. There will be four or five small bounces as you proceed from right to left. When the head and upper body have reached the left leg, inhale, and on exhalation bounce back toward the right. Repeat several times until the lower spine is loose and flexible; then proceed with forward-bending postures. For additional stretching of the hamstrings, this can also be performed with the toes pointing toward the ceiling.

STANDING HEAD-TO-KNEE POST

BENEFITS: Increases spinal flexibility • Improves posture • Reduces abdominal fat

PRECAUTIONS: Use caution if you have a bad back • Not for those with high or low blood pressure • Avoid if you have a hiatal hernia

DIRECTIONS: Stand erect, inhale, and extend the arms over the head and interlock thumbs. The upraised arms are touching the ears and remain in contact throughout the exercise. Exhale slowly, and bend forward from the thigh joints, bringing the forehead to the knee and locking the hands around the back of the ankles. Hold for as long as comfortable. Repeat several times.

Standing Head-to-Knee Post

RISHI'S POSTURE

BENEFITS: Counteracts body's imbalance or lopsidedness • Reduces waistline • Provides spinal flexibility • Promotes balance, grace, poise, and flexibility

DIRECTIONS: Stand erect with feet slightly apart, arms straight out in front of you at shoulder level, palms down, with thumbs hooked together. Keep the bottom half of your body facing forward, as you slowly turn the upper body and arms to the left as far as they will go. You will feel an intense stretching in the waist and back as you make this corkscrew-type twist. From this position, slowly bend down, and place the right hand on the back of the right ankle as shown. The left hand extends upward, and the eyes are focused on the back of the left hand. Hold for a count of ten. Slowly straighten up, bringing arms to original position, and repeat on the opposite side. Perform three times on each side.

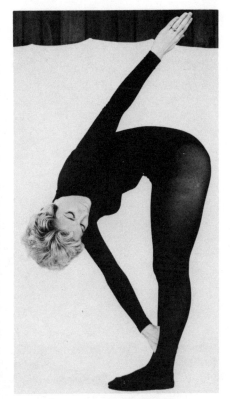

Rishi's Posture

HEAD-TO-KNEE POST

BENEFITS: Provides a natural follow-up for the Leg Pulls (page 122) and is also frequently performed before the Forward Bend as a warm-up for that posture • Eliminates tension from back and legs • Stretches the hamstrings

PRECAUTIONS: Do not go beyond the point of pain

DIRECTIONS: Sit on floor or mat with legs outstretched in front of you.

Bend the left knee, placing the sole of left foot against right inner thigh as shown. Inhale, and stretch the straightened arms toward the ceiling, then on exhalation slowly bend forward, grasping the leg as far down as you can without straining. Without allowing the back of the leg to lift from the floor, bring your forehead as close as you can to the right knee. Hold motionless for a count of ten. Repeat three times with each leg. Increase the holding time gradually until you can remain in the position for one minute, and then perform the posture only once. When you become more flexible, point the toe toward the ceiling; when this can be done easily, try the posture with the left foot on top of the right thigh in Half Lotus posture.

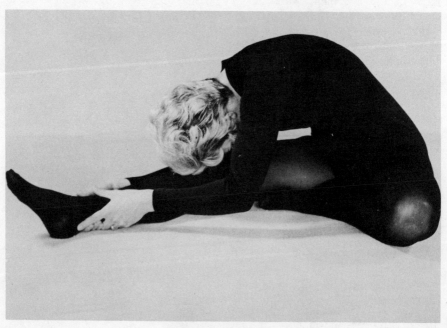

Head-to-Knee Post

WHEEL

BENEFITS: Strengthens the entire body • Provides spinal flexibility • Firms legs and thighs

PRECAUTIONS: Bypass this one if you have a back problem

DIRECTIONS: Lie on your back, bend knees, and place feet flat on the floor twelve to eighteen inches apart and as close as possible to the buttocks. Place palms flat on floor at about ear level with fingers pointing toward your shoulders. Now arch your back, and raise buttocks off the floor. Continue arching the spine while pushing with the arms until the entire torso is off the floor as shown. Hold for a count of ten; repeat three times. Increase the time posture is

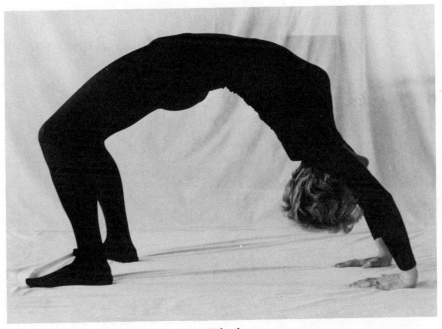

Wheel

held until you can maintain it for one minute. Very advanced students, particularly those with strong backs, may raise one leg until it is parallel to the floor while doing this posture, but proceed carefully. Also, as you become more advanced, work toward inching the hands and feet closer together while in the posture.

POSE OF A CHILD
(Folded Leaf or Fetal Position)

BENEFITS: Provides a good resting position after positions that flex the spine backward and those that activate the thigh muscles • Improves complexion

PRECAUTIONS: None

DIRECTIONS: Assume a position on hands and knees, lower the buttocks to rest on the lower legs, and place the forehead on the floor.

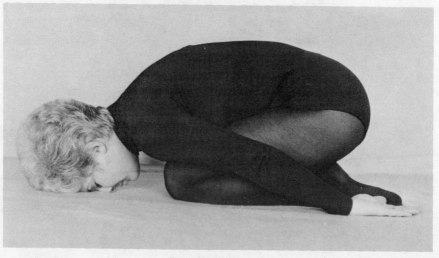

Pose of a Child

Relax completely, and let the arms lie limply by the sides, palms up. Hold the pose, inhaling and exhaling deeply, until the muscles and the breathing return to normal.

TRIANGLE

BENEFITS: Reduces fat around waistline • Sculptures legs and thighs • Provides a powerful and unusual stretch for the spine

PRECAUTIONS: Proceed cautiously if you have a back problem

DIRECTIONS: ، Assume a stance with your feet two to three feet apart. Slowly raise your arms straight out at the sides to shoulder level, palms down. Inhale, and slowly bend to the left until you can grasp left ankle with your left hand. Bend directly to the side and not to the front. The right arm swings in a wide arc over

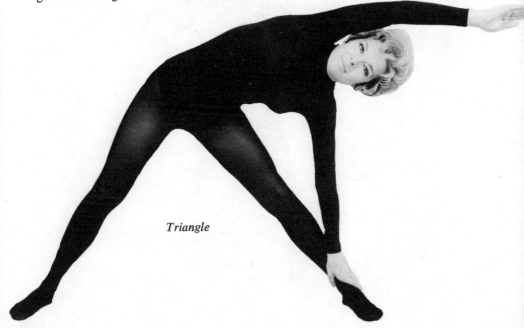

Triangle

your head until the inside of the elbow is alongside your ear. Your right arm should be parallel to the floor with palm down. Hold for a count of ten; exhale as you return to the original stance. Perform the identical movements to the right side; repeat three times on each side.

TRIANGLE—TWISTING VARIATION

BENEFITS: Provides a unique twisting action for the spine • Whittles the waistline • Tones up abdominal organs

PRECAUTIONS: Use caution if you have a back problem

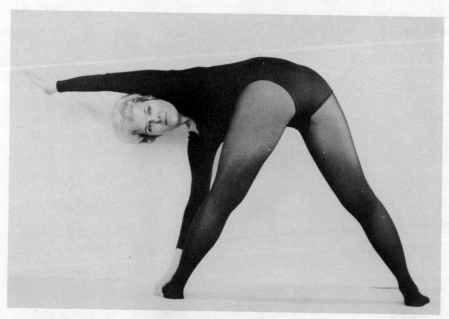

Triangle—Twisting Variation

DIRECTIONS: Assume a stance with feet two to three feet apart. Extend the straightened arms to the sides at shoulder level, palms down. Twist the upper body as far as possible to the left. Then grasp left foot with right hand while bringing left arm to a position alongside the ear and parallel to the ground. Hold for thirty seconds, and repeat on the other side. Perform three times on each side at first. When the posture can be maintained easily, perform it only once, and hold for increasingly longer periods of time, up to two minutes.

SHOULDER PULLS

BENEFITS: Releases accumulated tension in shoulders and upper back • Improves posture • Helps prevent bursitis and the formation of calcium deposits in the shoulder joints • Helps correct minor spinal misalignments

PRECAUTIONS: None

DIRECTIONS: With your right hand, reach over your right shoulder until the elbow is pointing straight up toward the ceiling. With the left arm close to the rib cage, bring the left hand behind the back, and try to grasp the right hand as shown. Now pull up with the right hand, then down with the left. Repeat several times until back and shoulders feel loosened up. Reverse the position so that the left elbow points to the ceiling, and repeat. Because our bodies develop onesidedly, you will find it easier to reach on one side than on

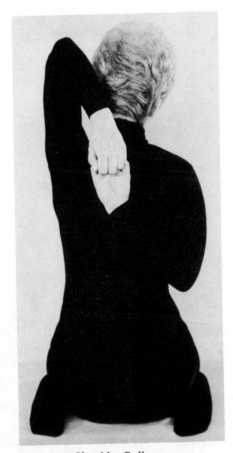

Shoulder Pulls

the other, or you may not be able to reach at all. For those unable to reach at all, use a handkerchief or a short piece of rope until the muscles become stretched enough to allow the hands to meet.

BLADE

BENEFITS: Much the same as the Shoulder Pulls except they are accomplished through horizontal movements and the Shoulder Pulls are vertical • Improves bustline through strengthening the pectoral muscles

DIRECTIONS: Sit or stand, and extend arms straight out to the side at shoulder level. Pull the shoulder blades together as though you are trying to pinch a dime between them. Do not initiate this movement by moving the arms back, but let the muscles do the work. The arms and shoulders will come back automatically. Repeat as many times as is needed to eliminate tension.

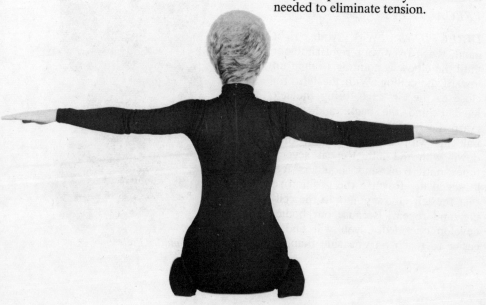

Blade

SHOULDER FLEXING

BENEFITS: Relieves tension in neck, back, and shoulders • Increases lung capacity • Prevents dowager's hump • Warms the body up for more advanced postures

DIRECTIONS: Sit in Half or Full Lotus or any cross-legged position—or stand if you prefer. Place the fingertips on the shoulders as shown.

Step 1: Inhale, then as you exhale, drop the head to the chest, and bring the elbows together in front of the body.

Step 2: Inhale, raising the head up and back while the elbows are drawn back as though trying to bring them together behind the back. Establish a rhythm, inhaling and exhaling, and repeat ten to fifteen times.

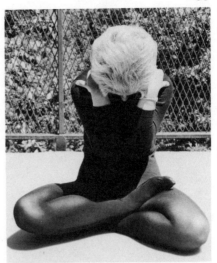

Shoulder Flexing—Step 1

SHOULDER MASSAGE

BENEFITS: Eases tension in upper back and shoulder blades

DIRECTIONS: Lie on back with feet eighteen to twenty-four inches apart. Place the fingertips on top of the shoulders at the outer edge close to the arm juncture. Inhale, and bring

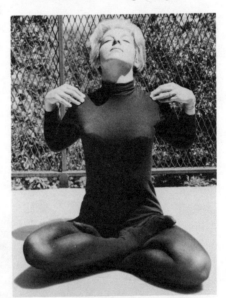

Shoulder Flexing—Step 2

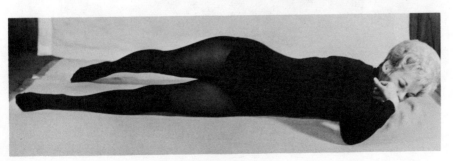

Shoulder Massage

the right elbow across to touch the floor on the left side of the body, rolling the shoulder-blade area and upper back firmly across the mat as you do so. Both heels remain on the floor, providing the necessary balance. Exhale, and roll to the other side, touching the left elbow to the floor on the right side of the body. Continue rolling back and forth until the shoulder blades feel relaxed.

DEER POSTURE

BENEFITS: Loosens lower back and hamstrings • Firms the buttocks • Removes abdominal fat and massages internal organs

PRECAUTIONS: Approach cautiously if you have a bad back • Avoid this if you have a hiatas hernia

DIRECTIONS: Sit with legs outstretched, toes pointed toward the

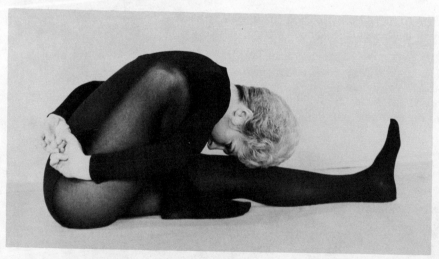

Deer Posture

ceiling. Bend the right knee, and bring heel up as close to the buttocks as possible. Bend forward, bring the forehead down to touch the left knee, and at the same time bring the hands together behind your back, encircling the upraised right knee. Try to hold for thirty seconds, breathing deeply. Repeat on other side. You may gradually increase your time in this posture, up to two minutes.

CAMEL (PELVIC STRETCH)

BENEFITS: Increases spinal flexibility • Firms and shapes hips and thighs • Removes fat deposits from upper legs and abdomen • Corrects round shoulders and improves posture

PRECAUTIONS: Do not attempt this if you have a back problem

DIRECTIONS: Assume a kneeling position with legs slightly separated. Relax a moment. Inhale, and arch the spine, raising the pelvis, and reach back to grasp the heels of the ankles. Keep your elbows straight, and let your head droop backward as shown. You will have a stretched feeling in the muscles of neck, chest, waist, abdomen, and thighs. Hold for a count of ten; exhale and relax. Repeat three times. Following this posture, relax in the Pose of a Child shown on page 128.

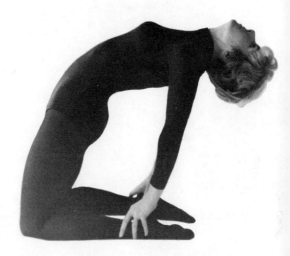

Camel (Pelvic Stretch)

Variation #1: If this posture seems too difficult at first, you may modify it by sitting back on your heels, keeping your arms straight with palms on floor at your sides slightly

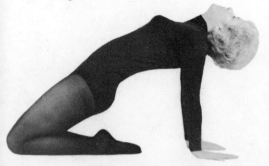

Camel—Variation #1

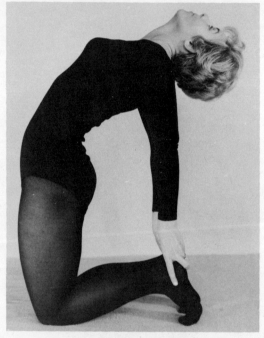

Camel—Variation #2

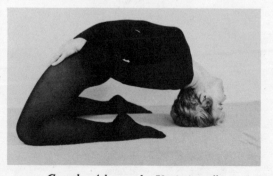

Camel—Advanced—Variation #3

behind your buttocks, then arching the spine.

Variation #2 is also an easier modification of the Camel. To perform this, flex the toes as shown, then arch the spine as you reach back to grasp the heels.

CAMEL—ADVANCED—VARIATION #3

BENEFITS: Provides a challenge for the advanced student • Strengthens back muscles and increases spinal flexibility • Greatly strengthens and stretches the thigh muscles

PRECAUTIONS: Everyone should approach this posture with extreme caution • Those with back problems should avoid it

DIRECTIONS: Kneel with knees spread as far apart as comfortably possible and with the hands resting lightly on fronts of thighs. Arch the back as much as possible, then bend the knees to slowly lower the body, proceeding only as long as you are in complete control. At first, it may be a good idea to place a pillow at the spot where your head will be. After the head touches the floor, slowly raise the body to its original position, then assume the Pose of a Child, which will provide the necessary reverse curving of the spine.

THREE-POSITION SIDE STRETCH

BENEFITS: Reduces waistline flabbiness • Firms the entire side of the body • Beneficially stretches the spine

PRECAUTIONS: Be careful if you have a back problem

DIRECTIONS: Stand erect with feet together, arms straight over the head, palms together. Inhale, and bend sideways from the hip just slightly. Hold for a count of ten. Exhale, return to original position, and repeat on the other side. Repeat again, bending slightly farther to the side. Repeat on the other side, and return to original position. Now inhale, and bend as far to the side as possible. Hold for a count of ten. Repeat on the other side. Be sure to bend to the side and not forward.

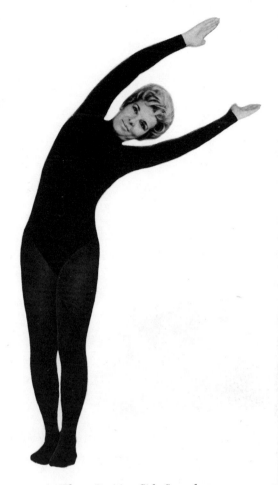

Three-Position Side Stretch

LEG ELONGATOR

BENEFITS: Eases some cases of backache

PRECAUTIONS: Do not hold longer than a count of sixty

DIRECTIONS: Lying in bed or on a flat, firm surface, place feet together, anklebone to anklebone. Without

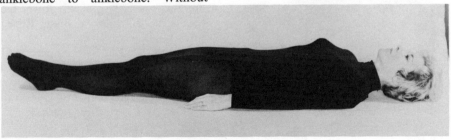

Leg Elongator

lifting it, stretch the right leg as though you were trying to elongate the leg. The right leg will now be one-half inch to one inch longer than the left. Hold for a count of thirty, and return to original position. Repeat with the left leg. This stretching of the spinal column is very effective and will be felt from the hip down. You can gradually work up to a count of sixty with each leg, but this is the maximum. You may perform the exercise morning and night if you wish.

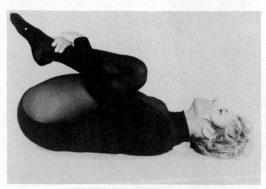

Wind-Relieving Posture—Step 1

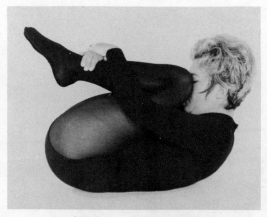

Wind-Relieving Posture—Step 2

WIND-RELIEVING POSTURE

BENEFITS: Relieves flatulence (about two hours after performance of the posture) • Eliminates constipation • Strengthens abdominal, neck, and back muscles • Improves complexion

PRECAUTIONS: If you have a weak back, place your hands beneath the small of the back while lowering legs • If you have high blood pressure, avoid this exercise

DIRECTIONS: Step 1: Lie flat on floor or mat. Inhale, and draw knees up tightly against chest as shown. Retain breath, and hold for a count of ten. Straighten knees, and use abdominal muscles to slowly lower feet to the floor while exhaling. Repeat three times.

Step 2: Repeat Step 1, except lift the head, and touch forehead to knees as you count to ten. Lower head to floor, and exhale as you slowly lower feet. Repeat three times.

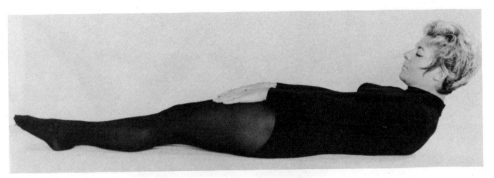

Wind-Relieving Posture—Step 3

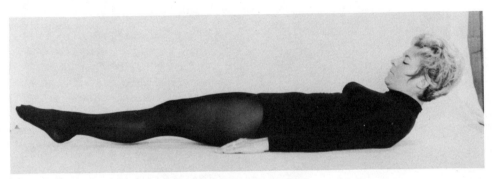

Wind-Relieving Posture—Step 4

Step 3: Lying flat on floor, place palms down flat on the fronts of thighs. Inhale, and raise the head to look at toes, keeping shoulders on the floor. As you raise the head, the hands automatically slide down toward knees. Hold for a count of ten; exhale as you lower head. Repeat three times.

Step 4: Inhale, and raise head as in Step 3, and at the same time raise the heels one inch off the floor. Hold for a count of ten, then lower head and heels while exhaling. Repeat three times.

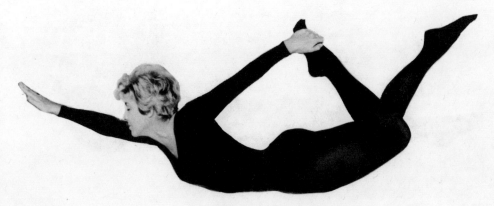

Half-Bow Half-Boat

HALF-BOW HALF-BOAT

BENEFITS: Tests your ability to concentrate while providing an excellent all-purpose stretch for the spine and legs

PRECAUTIONS:. Approach cautiously if you have a back problem

DIRECTIONS: Lie flat on stomach. Bend left knee, and reach back with left hand to grasp left ankle. The right leg remains flat, and the right arm is stretched out in front of the body. Relax completely for a second. Inhale, and push left foot as though trying to pull the ankle away from the hand. This creates tension and results in an arching of the spine. At the same time the right arm and leg are raised as shown. Hold for a count

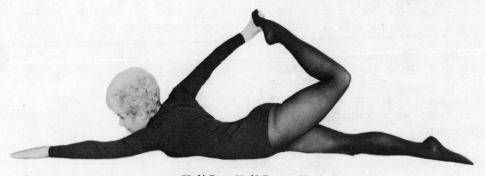

Half-Bow Half-Boat—Variation

of ten; exhale and relax, lying flat. Reverse the posture, performing the "bow" portion on the right side and the "boat" on the left. Repeat three times on each side, alternating sides.

Variation: Lie on your stomach. Grasp the left foot with the right hand while the left arm and right leg remain on the floor. Inhale, and bring the joined hand and foot up as high as you can; hold for a count of ten. Change position to grasp the right foot with the left hand, and repeat; perform three times on each side, alternating right and left sides. When this can be performed easily, try raising the arm and leg that were previously lying flat, as in the Half-Bow Half-Boat shown above.

HIDDEN LOTUS

BENEFITS: Yoga has many benefits—some that can be measured and evaluated, and some that are obvious only to those who experience them. This posture well illustrates the link between mind and body. It strengthens the hip joints and will give you a real mental lift.

PRECAUTIONS: Do not hold this posture for more than thirty seconds if you have varicose veins

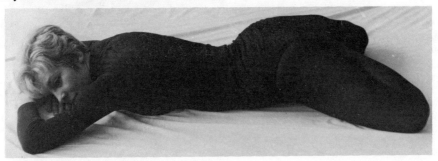

Hidden Lotus

DIRECTIONS: Assume the Full Lotus posture shown on page 112. Using the hands for balance, rise up on the knees, and come forward until you are lying on your stomach. Rest your head on folded arms, and keep thighs as flat as possible against the floor. Breathe deeply, and retain the posture as long as is comfortable. You will eventually be able to maintain this position for four to five minutes.

LYING LEG STRETCH

BENEFITS: Eliminates "saddlebags" • Firms and trims inner thigh

PRECAUTIONS: Don't overdo this one

DIRECTIONS: In performing this posture you will be drawing a half circle with the leg. Lie on floor or mat with hands at sides and legs straight. Slowly cross the right leg over the left. Keep the shoulders flat on the floor and the right leg close to the floor. Continue moving the right leg, with knee straight, until you reach the position shown. At this point you

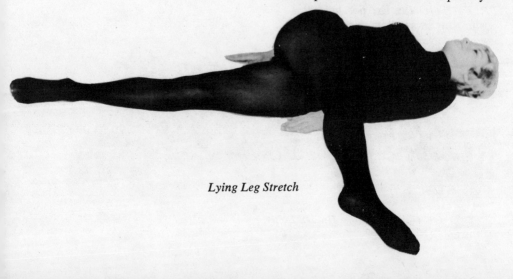

Lying Leg Stretch

have drawn a quarter circle with the toe. Now raise the right leg until the toe points to the ceiling. Continue lowering the leg to the floor on the other side. The leg should extend at approximately a 90° angle from the body, which will provide an intense stretch for the inner thigh and the thigh joint. This lifting motion marks the diameter of the half circle. Now bring the toe back to the starting point, and without pausing continue until you have made three half circles with the right leg. Repeat the same movements with the left leg.

SPINE STRETCHER

BENEFITS: Stretches and strengthens the back • Provides a unique twisting action for the spine • Develops control

PRECAUTIONS: Not for those with bad backs

DIRECTIONS: Lie on back with arms extended out from sides at shoulder level, palms flat on floor. Inhale, and slowly raise both legs until they are at right angles to the body, toes pointing toward the ceiling. Without pausing, and on exhalation, bring the legs down toward the left hand. Hold for a moment, inhale, and bring the legs back up until toes point toward the ceiling. On exhalation bring legs down toward the right hand. The shoulders remain flat on the floor throughout. Perform five times on each side. Don't be discouraged if you can't get toes close to your hand at first.

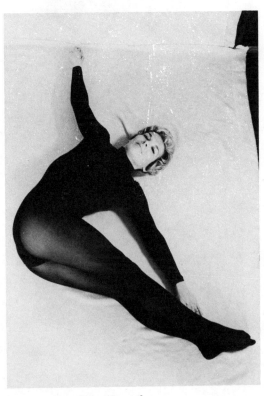

Spine Stretcher

SCORPION

In yoga progress is more important than perfection. A posture that is finally achieved after many failures, or one that has taken a long time to master, has more value than one effortlessly assumed. The Scorpion is a very advanced posture and one that I tried three times a day for more than a year before mastering. It should be attempted only after the Headstand is easily and effortlessly maintained. Remember that any posture proving difficult is attempted three times during an exercise period and abandoned until the next day. This approach eliminates our culture's demand for instant perfection. The sense of adequacy achieved when the posture is finally mastered is a step toward a more mature approach to life.

BENEFITS: Stretches almost all the muscles in the body, particularly those of the lower back • Improves circulation • Provides a tremendous psychological lift

DIRECTIONS: Assume the yoga Headstand (page 116). From this position slowly bend the knees and arch the spine accordingly to maintain balance. Unclasp the fingers, and place palms flat on the floor a comfortable distance apart. The body's weight is now balanced on the arms and hands. Slowly raise the head while maintaining balance. Hold for as long as comfortable.

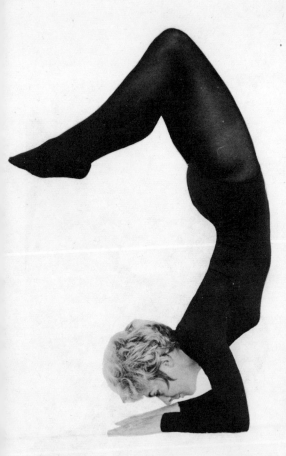

Scorpion

ANGLE BALANCE

BENEFITS: Improves balance • Stretches hamstrings • Firms abdominal muscles

PRECAUTIONS: None

DIRECTIONS: Sit on floor or mat with the knees bent and the soles of the feet together and flat on the floor. Grasp the ankles, and slowly straighten both elbows and knees to assume the position shown. Once the position is assumed, the body has a tendency to roll over backward. Concentrate on remaining balanced on the buttocks for a count of ten, increasing the time gradually. When this has been mastered, perform the variation in which the toes are grasped, providing a more intense stretch for the hamstrings. When this variation can be easily maintained, bring both legs together in front of your body, then try touching the forehead to the knees while maintaining balance.

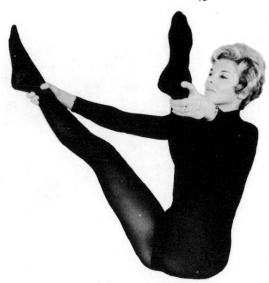

Angle Balance

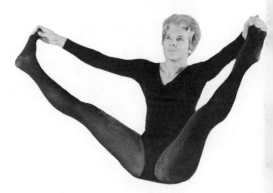

Angle Balance—Variation

ARCH POSTURE

BENEFITS: Strengthens spine and back muscles • Firms legs and thighs • Tones up abdominal organs and removes abdominal fat

DIRECTIONS: Lie on back with arms outstretched, palms down. The knees are bent and heels close to the buttocks, heels eighteen to twenty-four inches apart. Inhale, and slowly raise the buttocks and then the back off the mat, one vertebra at a time. When the body is lifted as high as possible, as shown on page 146, hold for a count of ten, and exhale while

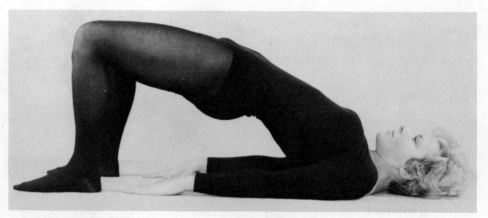

Arch Posture

slowly lowering the body back to the mat. When the body is again on the mat, press the small of your back against the mat, pull your stomach in, and hold, without inhaling, for a count of ten. Repeat three times.

ARCH POSTURE— PELVIC TILT VARIATION

This variation looks exactly like the Arch Posture, but the concentration is different.

BENEFITS: Probably the best exercise there is for relieving back problems (A chiropractor in one of my classes said that if the posture ever became common knowledge, he would be out of business.) • Firms legs and thighs • Removes abdominal fat • Improves concentration

DIRECTIONS: Lie on back with arms outstretched, palms down. Knees are bent and heels close to the buttocks, heels eighteen to twenty-four inches apart. After assuming this position, the pelvis is tilted upward. While maintaining this pelvic tilt, inhale, and slowly raise the buttocks and then the back off the mat, one vertebra at a time. The important thing to remember is to keep the pelvic tilted throughout the entire exercise. When the body is lifted as high as possible, hold for a count of ten; exhale, and slowly lower the body, one vertebra at a time, maintaining the pelvic tilt. Repeat three times.

ONE-LEG STAND

BENEFITS: Improves balance and posture • Provides a good overall stretch, particularly for legs, arms, and shoulders

DIRECTIONS: Stand erect with weight evenly distributed on both feet. Bend the left knee, and reach back and grasp the left foot with the left hand. Stretch the right arm toward the sky, palm up. Inhale, and stretch the left leg as far back and up as you can while maintaining balance. Try to remain in balance and motionless, inhaling and exhaling deeply, for as long as possible. Repeat on the other leg.

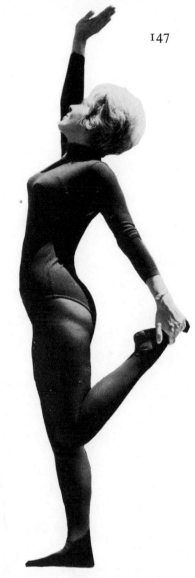

One-Leg Stand

One-Leg Stand—Variation

Variation: Repeat the above directions for assuming the One-Leg Stand, then on an exhalation bend forward as shown, trying to pull the left foot up as high as possible while maintaining balance. Try to remain in balance and motionless, inhaling and exhaling deeply, for as long as possible. Repeat on the other leg.

SUPINE PELVIC

BENEFITS: Provides a good counter-stretch following the Shoulder Stand • Firms the thighs and chin area • Eliminates constipation • Beneficially affects the pituitary, pineal, thyroid, and adrenal glands • Tones the female reproductive system, the abdominal muscles, and the nervous system

PRECAUTIONS: If you have a hyperactive thyroid, do not hold this posture longer than thirty seconds • Those with a back problem should approach this posture carefully

DIRECTIONS: On floor or mat, sit back on the heels, keeping the legs

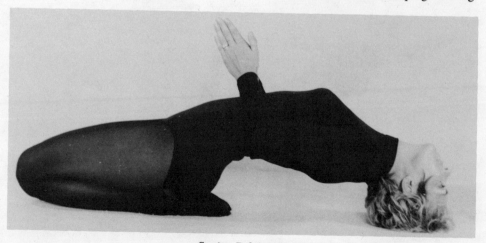

Supine Pelvic

together. Lean back on the elbows, arching the back, and place crown of head on the floor. The hands are positioned in an attitude of prayer as shown. Hold the pose, inhaling and exhaling slowly and deeply, as long as is comfortable, up to three minutes.

SUPINE PELVIC—VARIATION

BENEFITS: Firms the thighs • Calms the nervous system due to the rhythmic breathing employed • Stretches knees and spine

PRECAUTIONS: Avoid this if you have any knee problem

DIRECTIONS: Sit with buttocks on the floor between the legs. Using the arms for support, slowly lower the torso to the mat, trying to keep the back as flat as possible. Place the arms in the position shown, and

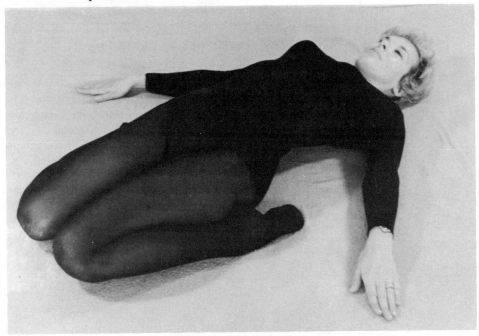

Supine Pelvic—Variation

slowly inhale to a count of six while raising the straightened arms to the sides along the floor until they are parallel and pointing over the head. When the arms are nearly parallel, turn the hands over so the palms are up. Hold for a count of three, and exhale to a count of six while bringing the straightened arms down in an arc over the body until they are in the original position. Remain in this position for a count of three, then repeat the entire exercise six times.

TWIST VARIATIONS

BENEFITS: These three spinal twist variations all relieve tightness and spasm in the back and shoulder-blade area and increase spinal flexibility. However, there are subtle differences in each, depending on individual proportions, which must be experienced kinesthetically to be fully appreciated.

PRECAUTIONS: Be careful if you have a back problem

DIRECTIONS: Variation #1: Sit with legs outstretched. Bend the right knee, and place right heel under left hip. Now bend left knee, and position left ankle alongside the right knee as shown. Lean forward, stretch left arm around left knee, and join your hands behind your back. Those familiar with the standard full Spinal Twist will notice that it utilizes the opposite arm from this variation. Inhale

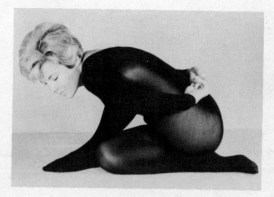

Twist—Variation #1

deeply, and feel the intense stretching along the left side of the back. Hold for a count of ten, and exhale. Repeat three times on each side, alternating sides. When you have become adept at this pose, you may perform it only once on each side, holding for a longer period of time, up to two minutes.

Variation #2 (the Pretzel): Sit with legs outstretched. Bend left knee, and place left foot under the right upper thigh. Place right foot flat on floor with right ankle beside the left knee as shown. Place left arm under right knee as shown, and join the hands. Twist upper body around to the right; inhale, hold for a count of ten, exhale, and relax. Repeat three times on each side, alternating sides. As you become more flexible, you may perform it only once on each side, holding for a longer period of time, up to two minutes.

Variation #3 (Rishi's Twist): Sit in Half Lotus posture with left foot placed on top of right thigh. Stretch left arm behind you, and grasp toes of left foot in the left hand. Twist upper body to the extreme left, and place the right hand under left knee with fingers pointing toward your body. In addition to the spine, this variation also beneficially affects the wrists, providing increased flexibility. Inhale, hold the posture for a count of ten, exhale, and relax. Repeat three times on each side, alternating sides. As you become more adept at the posture, you may perform it only once on each side, holding for a longer period of time, up to two minutes.

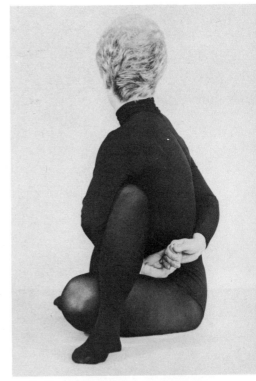

Twist—Variation #2 (the Pretzel)

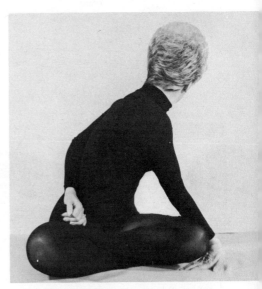

Twist—Variation #3 (Rishi's Twist)

BRIDGE

The Bridge is an intermediate-to-advanced posture that teaches control. While many postures are difficult to hold or maintain, the primary difficulty of the Bridge lies in getting into it in a controlled manner. Once in the position, it is relatively easy to hold. The second and final challenge comes in trying to come out of the Bridge gracefully.

BENEFITS: Strengthens back muscles • Provides proper counteracting bend for the spine following the Shoulder Stand

PRECAUTIONS: Not recommended for those with a back problem

DIRECTIONS: Assume the Shoulder Stand posture. If you are doubtful about your ability to execute this posture, you may begin it from the Half Shoulder Stand, which is less difficult. Change the hand position so that the thumbs face each other on your back and the fingers are in front of your rib cage. Be sure that your elbows are close together and perpendicular to the floor—they form the support for your bridge. Bend the left knee, and bring it close to your forehead for balance. Then lower the right leg to the floor. Extend the left

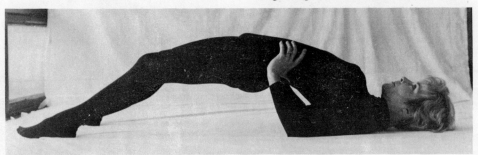

Bridge

leg out beside the right. The feet are flat on the floor and extended so that the knees are nearly straight and the body forms an arch as shown. Hold for ten seconds to begin, gradually increasing the time until you can hold it for two minutes. To come out of the Bridge, raise one leg at a time, and return to the Shoulder Stand. Repeat with the other leg. With practice it is possible to move from the Shoulder Stand into the Bridge and back again easily and gracefully. When you become more advanced, you can bring both legs down together. To do this, bend both knees, and bring them close to your forehead. Bend quickly so that you roll your back over your thumbs and bring both feet to the floor.

SIDE LEG RAISE

BENEFITS: Firms inner thighs • Trims outer thigh bulges • Reduces the waistline

PRECAUTIONS: None

DIRECTIONS: Lie on floor or mat with one arm supporting the head and the other placed in front of you for balance. Raise the upper leg sideways as high as possible as in Step 1.

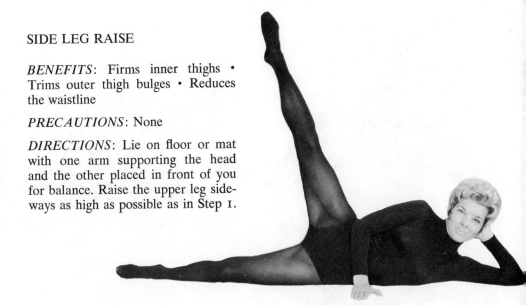

Side Leg Raise—Step 1

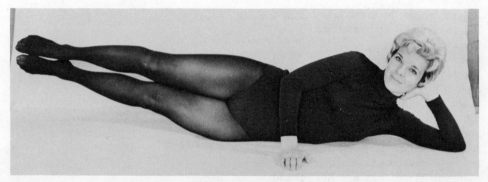

Side Leg Raise—Step 2

Be sure the raising motion is sideways and not forward. Hold for a count of ten, and slowly lower the leg. Now lift both legs together as high as possible sideways as in Step 2, and hold for a count of ten. Repeat three times, then turn to the other side and perform three times on that side.

POSE OF A FROG

BENEFITS: Increases flexibility in ankle and knee joints

PRECAUTIONS: Avoid this if you have had knee injuries or problems

DIRECTIONS: Kneel on floor or mat, keeping the feet together. Now spread the knees as far apart as possible, keeping the big toes touching. You will actually be sitting in front of your feet. Use the thumbs somewhat as a shoehorn to push the heels away from the body and provide more sitting space. When the heels have been pushed as far as they will go, place the hands on the knees, and hold the position as long as is comfortable, up to two minutes.

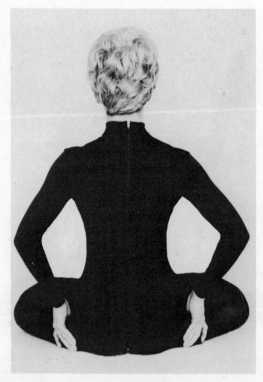

Pose of a Frog

TORTOISE

BENEFITS: Young children love the feeling of accomplishment gained through yoga. My then five-year-old daughter, Page, was elated over mastering the Tortoise, which she demonstrates. Only a handful of my adult students can do this demanding posture, which insures spinal flexibility and tones up hips and thighs.

DIRECTIONS: Sitting on floor or mat, spread legs as far apart as possible. Bend forward from the thigh joints, and place arms under legs as shown. The head and shoulders are resting on the floor in front.

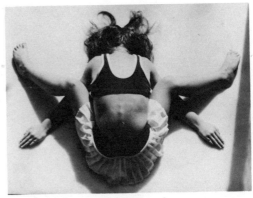

Tortoise

KNEELING POSE

The Kneeling Pose has attracted the critical attention of the medical press as the cause of an injury known as "yoga foot drop." Performed by sitting back on the heels as shown, the Kneeling Pose is normally held for short periods of time, which is not dangerous. When it is maintained longer during chanting or meditation, it places great pressure on the vulnerable peroneal nerve, which winds around the head of the fibula (outer leg bone) just below the knee, causing the feet to droop.

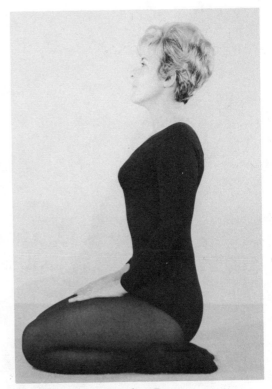

Kneeling Pose

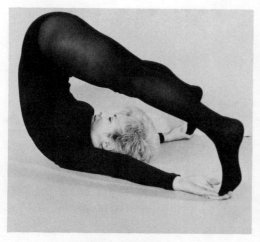

Plough—Legs Apart

PLOUGH—LEGS APART

BENEFITS: Stretches the cervical spine and increases circulation in this area • Firms the inner thighs and stretches the hamstrings

PRECAUTIONS: Be careful if you have a back problem

DIRECTIONS: From the Shoulder Stand posture, slowly bring the feet down to the floor over the head. Spread the legs apart as shown, then grasp the toes and remain in this position for as long as is comfortable, up to two minutes.

PLOUGH—WALKING TOES

BENEFITS: Provides an unusual stretch and twist for the spine • Improves muscular control

PRECAUTIONS: Be extra careful if you have a back problem

DIRECTIONS: Assume the Plough posture. Then slowly and in control move both feet as far as you can to the left. Hold for a moment in the extreme position, then move both feet as far as you can to the right. Repeat several times.

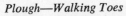

Plough—Walking Toes

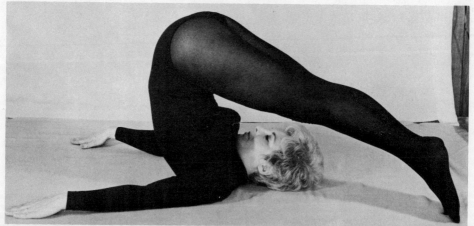

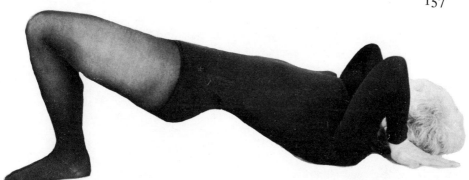

BACK PUSH-UP

Back Push-up

BENEFITS: Strengthens back, leg, arm, and abdominal muscles • Conditions the body for the more strenuous Wheel

DIRECTIONS: Lie on back with knees bent, heels close to the buttocks, and hands placed above the shoulders as shown, with fingers pointing away from the body. Inhale, and arch the lower body as high off the mat as possible. Hold for a count of ten; exhale, and lower the body back to the mat. Repeat three times.

CHEST EXPANSION—SEATED

BENEFITS: Increases lung capacity • Firms and develops the chest and bust • Prevents or improves dowager's hump • Eases tension in back and shoulder area • Improves posture

DIRECTIONS: Sit in Lotus, Half Lotus, or cross-legged position. Interlock the fingers behind your back at floor level or just above. Inhale, turn the interlocked fingers so the palms point away from you, and at the same time lift the arms as high as you can while pulling the shoulder blades together and looking up toward the ceiling. Hold for a count of ten, then

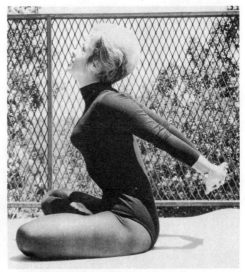

Chest Expansion—Seated

exhale, and drop the arms and the chin back to the starting position. Repeat three times.

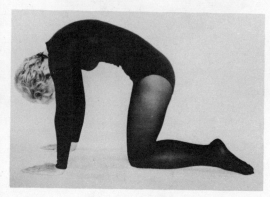

Cat Stretch—Step 1

CAT STRETCH

BENEFITS: Works kinks out of the spine • Stretches and strengthens the entire spine • Firms and trims the buttocks and legs

PRECAUTIONS: None

DIRECTIONS: Step 1: Kneel on hands and knees so that the back is parallel to the floor and the arms and legs resemble the legs of a table. Exhale, and slowly arch the back as shown, pulling the abdomen up toward the spine. Hold for a count of five.

Step 2: Now inhale as you flex the spine in the opposite direction, releasing the abdomen and stretching the neck to look toward the ceiling. Hold for a count of five.

Step 3: Arch the spine as in Step 1, and at the same time bring the knee up to touch the nose, or come as close as you can; hold for a count of five.

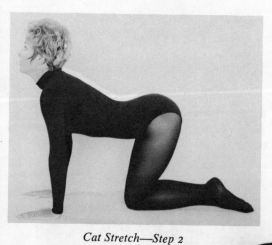

Cat Stretch—Step 2

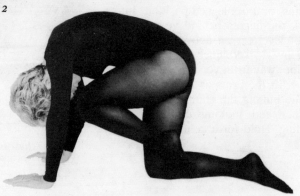

Cat Stretch—Step 3

Step 4: Repeat Step 2, and at the same time extend the leg back and up as far as you can for a count of five. Repeat several times on each side until the spine feels flexible.

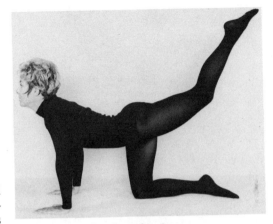

Cat Stretch—Step 4

CRESCENT MOON POSTURE

BENEFITS: Provides a powerful stretch for the entire body, particularly the legs and spine • Improves balance and posture

PRECAUTIONS: Be careful if you have a back problem

DIRECTIONS: Assume a position with the left knee on floor or mat, right leg bent at the knee and the foot flat on the floor. Extend left leg out behind the body as shown. Raise arms over the head, palms together. Bend right knee as much as possible while stretching up and back with the arms and upper body. Hold position for a count of ten, trying to stretch the body back as far as possible. Repeat three times with each leg. When you can easily maintain balance in this position, perform only once on each side, holding the posture for increasingly longer periods of time, up to two minutes.

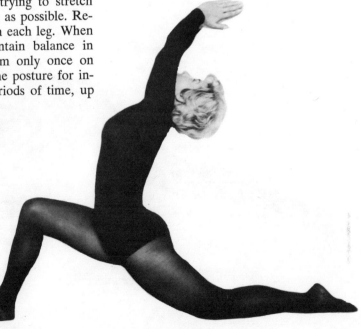

Crescent Moon Posture

DEEP LUNGE

BENEFITS: Firms and shapes legs • Trims flabby inner thighs • Conditions the legs for skiing through increased strength and pliability in legs and ankles • Improves balance

PRECAUTIONS: None

DIRECTIONS: Stand with feet as far apart as possible, the right toe pointing straight ahead and the left angled toward the left. The hands are clasped lightly behind your back. Inhale, and on exhalation bend the left knee sharply, and try to bring the forehead down to touch the floor beside your left foot. You will have to bring the trunk down beside your bent knee instead of over it. If you bend over the knee, it will prevent your getting any farther down. As you bend forward, the right leg remains straight and the right foot rolls sideward, stretching the muscles along the entire inside of the leg. Hold for a count of ten; repeat on other side. Bend in each direction three times.

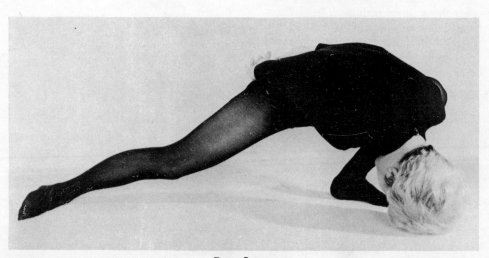

Deep Lunge

DEEP LUNGE—VARIATION

BENEFITS: Loosens the lower spine and stretches the hamstrings

DIRECTIONS: Stand with feet quite widespread and hands clasped behind your back for balance. Inhale, and on exhalation bend from the thigh joints, and bring the head down to touch one knee. Inhale as you return to the starting position, and on exhalation bring the forehead down to touch the other knee. Repeat three times on each side.

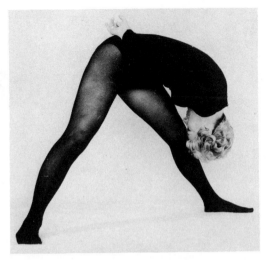

Deep Lunge—Variation

HINGE

BENEFITS: Strengthens weak abdominal muscles, a common cause of low-back pain

PRECAUTIONS: If your lower back is weak, support it with a small pillow during this exercise

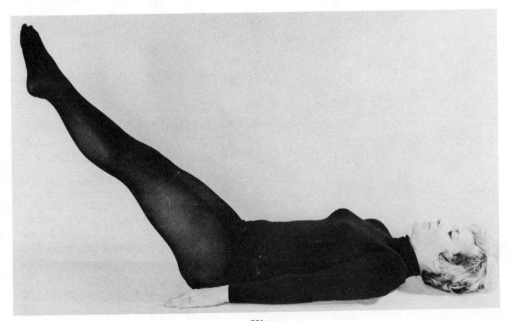

Hinge

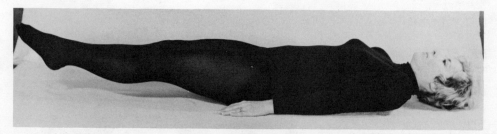

Rusty Hinge

DIRECTIONS: Lie on floor or mat; inhale, and slowly raise the legs, keeping the knees straight, until they are at right angles to the floor and the toes are pointing toward the ceiling. Slowly lower the legs until they are approximately halfway back to the floor as shown at bottom of page 106. Hold for a count of ten, then continue to lower the legs until they are a scant one-half inch off the floor, the Rusty Hinge position, and hold for a count of ten. Gradually increase the time that you can hold these two variations. Simple as these appear, they demand a great deal from abdominal muscles.

INCLINED PLANE

BENEFITS: Provides a natural follow-up for forward-bending postures • Strengthens arm and back muscles • Firms hips, stomach, and thighs

PRECAUTIONS: None

DIRECTIONS: Assume a sitting position on mat or floor. The arms are straight and placed on the floor, palms down, slightly behind the buttocks. Inhale, and raise the entire

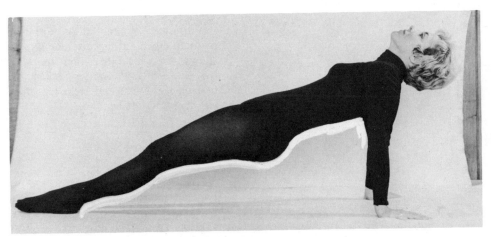

Inclined Plane

torso, the weight resting entirely on soles of feet and palms. Hold the posture, with the body stiff and the spine straight. Do not allow the body to sag in the middle. Hold for a count of ten, exhale, and lower the body to the original position. Repeat three times. Gradually increase the time the posture is held, and then perform it only once.

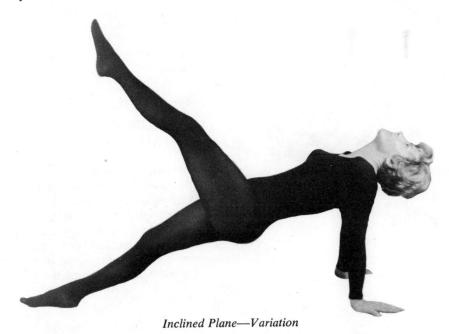

Inclined Plane—Variation

Variation: When the posture can be maintained easily, raise one leg, as shown, then the other; then try raising one arm and one leg, balancing first on right arm and right leg, then left arm and left leg, etc.

LYING TWIST

BENEFITS: Provides a corkscrew twisting motion for the spine • Relaxes the entire spine • Massages tension out of the shoulder area • Slims the waistline and trims the hips

PRECAUTIONS: None

DIRECTIONS: Lie on back with fingers interlaced and placed under the back of the neck. Bend knees, and place the soles of your feet as close to your buttocks as possible. Inhale, and on exhalation twist the knees to the left, keeping anklebones together, until left side of the leg touches the floor. Inhale as you bring the knees back up, and on exhalation lower the legs to the other side. The shoulders remain flat on the floor throughout the exercise. Repeat several times until the spine feels flexible.

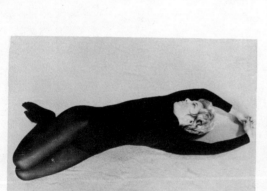

Lying Twist

LYING TWIST—VARIATION #1

Interlock the fingers, and extend the arms over the head as you press the spine against the floor. Inhale, and on exhalation slowly turn the head to the right as the legs are brought down on the left side. Inhale as you return to the original position, and on exhalation turn the head to

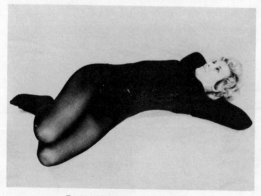

Lying Twist—Variation

the left and lower the legs to the right. This exercise is one continuous undulating motion and should be repeated until the spine feels free of tension.

LYING TWIST—
VARIATION #2
(Lucy's Posture)

Lying on back, place the sole of right foot just above the left knee. Grasp right knee with left hand and extend right arm to the side at shoulder level. Inhale, and on exhalation pull the right knee down to the floor on the left side of the body. At the same time, turn your head to the right. Repeat on the other side. Repeat several times, alternating sides.

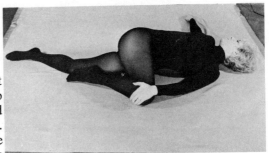

Lying Twist—Variation #2 (Lucy's Posture)

POSE OF A MOUNTAIN—
IN FULL LOTUS

BENEFITS: Eases tension in back and shoulder blades • Improves posture

PRECAUTIONS: Those with varicose veins should not hold the full lotus for more than thirty seconds

DIRECTIONS: Sit in Full Lotus posture if possible. If you have not yet mastered this, sit in Half Lotus, or cross-legged position. Hold the hands over the head and back as far as possible in an attitude of prayer. Be sure to keep the shoulders held well back; hold for as long as is comfortable, breathing deeply.

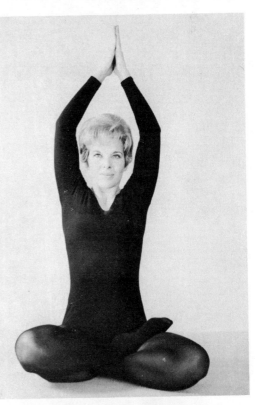

Pose of a Mountain in Full Lotus

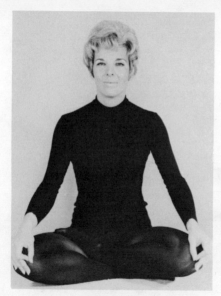

Half Lotus

HALF LOTUS

BENEFITS: Provides a meditative posture for those who have not mastered the Lotus.

DIRECTIONS: Sit with legs outstretched. Bend right knee and place right foot under left thigh. Now bend left knee, grasp left foot, and try to glide it on top of right thigh. Hold the posture as long as it is comfortable; then repeat with the other leg.

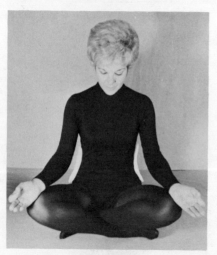

Easy Pose

EASY POSE

BENEFITS: The Easy Pose and the Ankle Lock Pose are two additional meditative postures that can be used by those who have not yet mastered the Lotus or the Half Lotus.

DIRECTIONS: Sit with spine straight. Fold the legs in front of you as shown. The hands rest on the knees and thumb and forefinger form a circle, with the thumb on top.

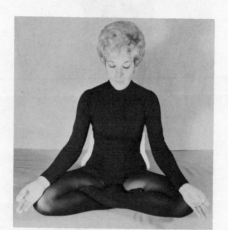

Ankle Lock Pose

ANKLE LOCK POSE

DIRECTIONS: Sit with legs crossed in front of you. Grasp the toes of the right foot and pull them up between the upper thigh and lower calf of left leg. Now tuck the toes of the left foot into the corresponding space on the right leg.

BACKWARD BEND

BENEFITS: Firms and develops the chest and bust • Stretches spine and increases flexibility • Prevents or improves dowager's hump, improves posture • Eases tension in back and shoulder area • Strengthens feet and ankles and imparts greater flexibility

PRECAUTIONS: If dizziness occurs, it indicates that blood flow through carotid arteries to brain is being restricted by extreme neck angle. Should this occur, assume the Pose of a Child, and rest until it passes; try with less head angle next time.

DIRECTIONS: Kneel with feet together and under you as shown. Place hands as far back as possible, with fingers pointing away from body. Allow head to droop backward. Inhale, and with an arching movement of back, raise body upward as far as you can without lifting buttocks. Hold for count of five, and exhale as you return to starting position. Repeat three times.

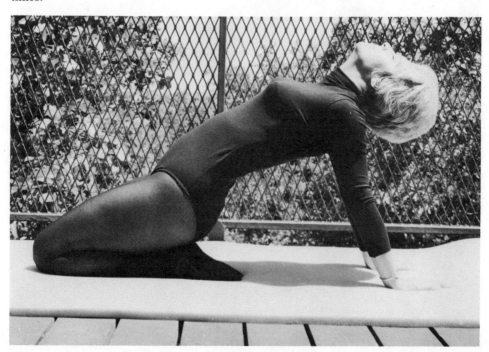

Backward Bend

PUMP IN HALF LOTUS

BENEFITS: Provides a good stretch for the spine and legs • Removes abdominal fat • Improves circulation • Provides beneficial massage for internal organs

PRECAUTIONS: Be careful if you have a back problem

DIRECTIONS: Assume the Shoulder Stand posture (page 97), with weight resting on the shoulders, upright body supported with both hands placed on back and toes pointed toward ceiling. Now bend left knee, and place left foot high on right thigh in Half Lotus posture. Inhale deeply, then exhale as you bring straightened right leg down so right toe touches floor over your head. Inhale as you bring right leg back to original posi-

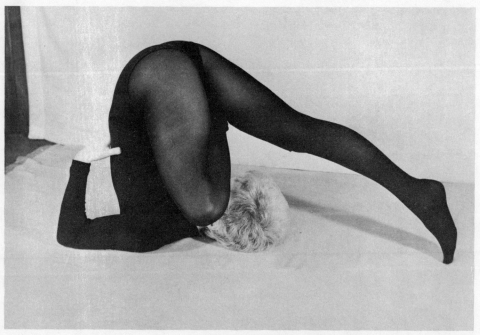

Pump in Half Lotus

tion. Change legs, repeating the same exercise with left leg. Perform three times with each leg, making sure breathing is done according to directions. If you have not yet mastered the Half Lotus, you may perform the Pump with straight legs. From Shoulder Stand, bring right leg down to touch floor on exhalation, inhale back up, and repeat with other leg. After touching floor twice with each leg, bring both legs down on exhalation, and without pausing raise them up on inhalation and repeat three times, trying to keep the trunk from moving.

EAGLE

BENEFITS: Firms legs, thighs, and hips • Improves balance • Teaches concentration

PRECAUTIONS: None

DIRECTIONS: Standing, lift right leg, and wrap the ankle around the left calf until toes of right foot are pointing frontward. Holding this position, entwine arms in front of chest, and lightly grasp nose with right thumb and forefinger. Bend forward, resting elbows on knee. Hold for as long as balance can be maintained. Repeat with other leg.

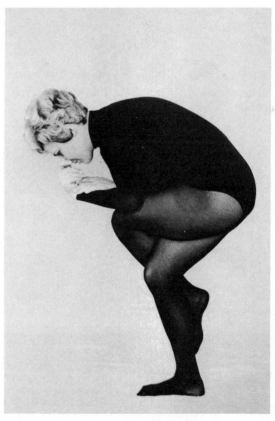

Eagle

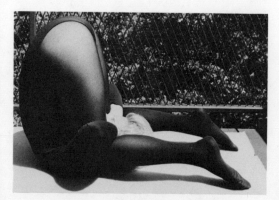

Choking Pose

CHOKING POSE

BENEFITS: Provides an excellent stretch for the entire spine • Stimulates the weight-regulating thyroid gland • Massages internal organs • Reduces abdominal fat

PRECAUTIONS: If you have a hyperactive thyroid, do not hold more than thirty seconds

DIRECTIONS: From the Plough posture (page 100), bend the knees, and bring them alongside the ears as shown. Then place the arms over the backs of the knees and the hands under the back of the neck. Breathe rhythmically, and remain in the posture as long as is comfortable, up to two minutes.

SIDE SLIP

BENEFITS: Whittles the waistline • Reduces hips, and slims and firms thighs • Improves posture • Gives the body grace in motion

PRECAUTIONS: None

DIRECTIONS: Assume a position standing on the knees with palms together and held over the back of the head as in Step 1. Slowly and gracefully lower the body to a sitting position to the right of the feet as shown in Step 2. The upper body bends in the opposite direction, giving the entire side an intense stretch. Then, again slowly and gracefully, lift the body with the thigh muscles, and place it on the other side of the feet, the upper body flexing in the opposite direction. This exercise is done

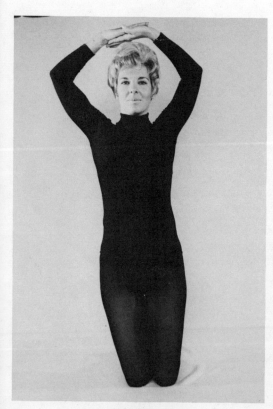

Side Slip—Step 1

slowly, gracefully, and rhythmically until the thigh muscles begin to feel fatigued, usually about ten times on each side. The hands remain in position throughout the exercise, and some students feel strain in the arms before the thigh muscles tire. Don't allow the body to sag forward, and keep the arms over the crown of the head throughout.

POSE OF A TREE

BENEFITS: Improves posture, balance, and poise

DIRECTIONS: Standing on a firm surface, bend one knee, and place the sole of that foot on the inside of the opposite thigh. Hold on to the back of a chair until you can balance on one foot. Place your palms together over the head as shown. The hands do not rest on the head, but are held above it. Also, be sure to keep the elbows back as far as possible, as this improves posture. Hold motionless for as long as comfortable, breathing slowly and rhythmically. Repeat on other foot. When you can hold the posture easily, try it with your eyes closed.

POSE OF A TREE—VARIATION

BENEFITS: Improves posture, balance, and poise

DIRECTIONS: Step 1: Standing on a firm surface, bend one knee, and place the foot on top of the opposite

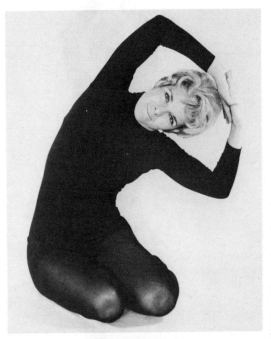

Side Slip—Step 2

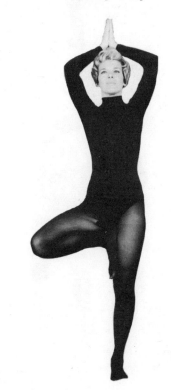

Pose of a Tree

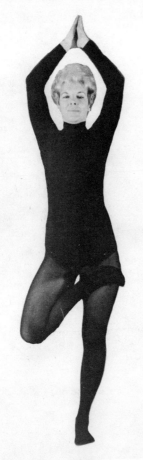

thigh as in Half Lotus posture. Place your palms together over your head as shown. To improve your posture, be sure to keep the elbows back as far as possible. Hold motionless for as long as comfortable, breathing slowly and rhythmically. Step 2: Inhale, and on exhalation bend forward while balancing on one leg, and place the hands on the floor as shown. Try to hold the posture without moving, up to one minute. Repeat on the other leg.

Pose of a Tree Variation—Step 1

STANDING FORWARD BEND— VARIATION

BENEFITS: Stretches and loosens hamstrings and lower back • Eases shoulder tension • Improves posture

DIRECTIONS: Stand with feet together, fingers interlocked behind your back, palms down. Inhale, step forward with one leg, and on exhalation bend forward from the thigh

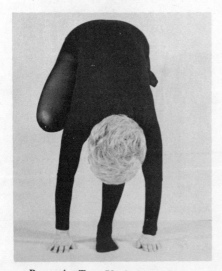

Pose of a Tree Variation—Step 2

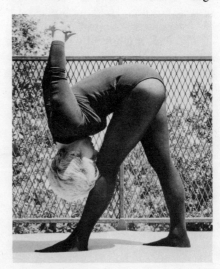

Standing Forward Bend

joints bringing the head to the knee as you bring the arms into the position shown with palms pointing toward the ceiling. Hold for a count of ten; repeat on the other side. Perform three times on each side.

Variation: Standing, interlock the fingers behind you, and stretch your spine upward as far as possible as you inhale. Slowly, exhaling, bend from the thigh joints, and raise the arms upward as shown. Inhaling, return to the original standing position, slightly arch the spine backward, and tilt the face skyward. Exhale as you repeat the forward bending; repeat several times until the spine feels relaxed and there is no tension between the shoulder blades.

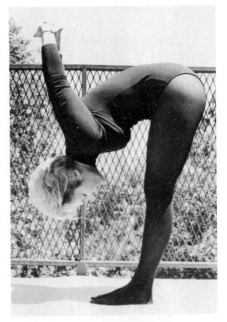

Standing Forward Bend—Variation

SQUATTING POSTURE

BENEFITS: Stretches and limbers stiff knees • Improves balance • Aids regularity • Conditions legs for skiing

PRECAUTIONS: Approach carefully if the knees have become stiff due to age, arthritis, or injury. Start by holding on to a doorknob, the back of a chair, or some other solid object. Gradually lower the body, maintaining balance, until the knees become more flexible.

DIRECTIONS: Stand with feet about a foot apart. Inhale deeply while rising up on tiptoe; hold for a few seconds. Slowly exhale while lowering the body by bending knees. In the extreme position you will be sitting back on the heels. Slowly raise the hands to the position shown. Concentrate on trying to bring the shoulder blades together, which is an aid

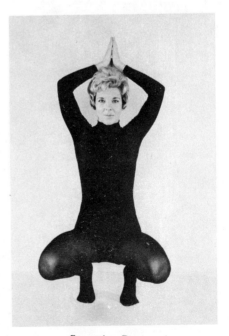

Squatting Posture

to correct posture. Hold the posture for a count of twenty. Lower hands, stand up slowly, take a deep breath, and relax. Repeat three times; when you can hold the posture for a minute or more, perform only once.

Butterfly

BUTTERFLY

BENEFITS: Firms inner thighs • Loosens thigh joints

DIRECTIONS: Sit on floor or mat with soles of the feet together. Grasp the toes firmly, and vigorously bounce the legs down toward the floor. Establish a rapid bouncing motion with the legs. This exercise is one of the few in yoga that utilizes fast repetitive motions. The pilot husband of one of my students encountered her doing the Butterfly and commented, "You'll never get it off the ground."

SWAN

BENEFITS: Step 1 strengthens and limbers up the spine, shoulders, pelvic area, and wrists • Step 2 aids the digestive organs, reduces abdominal fat, and strengthens the knees • The variation provides a counteracting flexing motion for the spine, strengthens wrists and forearms, and improves posture and coordination. This exercise is a good warm-up and is an instant invigorator.

PRECAUTIONS: Use care if you

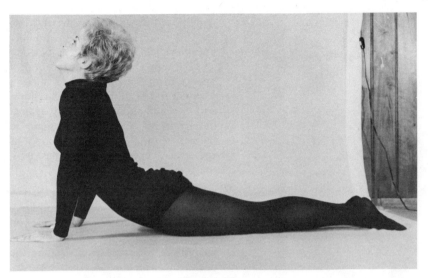

Swan—Step 1

have a back problem, or if your arms are extremely weak

DIRECTIONS: Step 1: This step resembles the Cobra except at the end when the elbows are straightened. Lie flat on stomach, palms flat on floor, the fingertips somewhat farther back from the top of shoulders than in the Cobra, and the elbows off the floor. Inhale deeply, and push down with hands until head, chest, and abdomen leave the floor and the elbows are straightened. Hold breath in this position as long as you comfortably can.

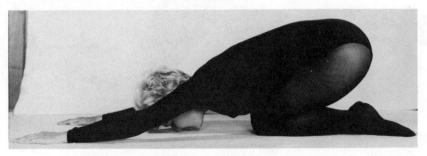

Swan—Step 2

Step 2: Keep hands where they are as you exhale, and bend the knees, which brings the buttocks to rest back on the heels. At the end of Step 2, arms are outstretched in front of you, forehead rests on the floor, and the abdomen is pressed against the fronts of the thighs. Remain in Step 2 without inhaling as long as you can. Repeat several times until the spine feels flexible.

Variation: Repeat Steps 1 and 2 above. After Step 2, inhale, and keep palms firmly against floor as you glide the body forward, supporting the weight with the arms, arching the back, and keeping the chest close to, but not touching, the floor. Continue this motion until you are again in the same position as you were at the end of Step 1, with the top half of the body off the floor and elbows straightened. Exhale as you repeat Step 2 and so on. Perform this exercise five or six times in continuous rhythmic motion.

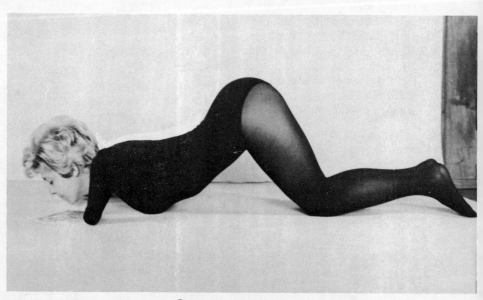

Swan—Variation

STANDING STAR

BENEFITS: Loosens up all parts of the body in preparation for more demanding postures • Step 1 works the kinks out of the lower spine • Step 2 eases tension from the upper back and shoulder blades • Steps 3 and 4 provide a necessary twisting motion for the spine and whittle the waistline • Step 5 flexes the entire spine in an opposite direction from Steps 1 and 2

PRECAUTIONS: If you have a bad back, perform Step 5 cautiously

DIRECTIONS: Step 1: Stand with feet eighteen to twenty-four inches apart. Bend the elbows, and place the left hand on upper right arm and the right hand on upper left arm as shown. Bend forward from the thigh joints, and gently bounce toward the floor five times.

Step 2: Extend both arms to the sides and back as far as you can, and with face forward, bounce the upper body down to a count of five.

Step 3: Raise the arms over the head, and place palms together. With the feet and lower body still facing forward, twist the arms and upper body to the right, and make rhythmic twisting movements to the count of five.

Step 4: Repeat Step 3, this time twisting the body to the left to a count of five.

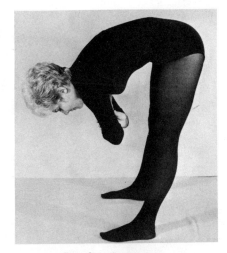

Standing Star—Step 1

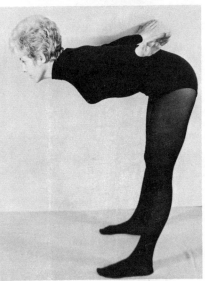

Standing Star—Step 2

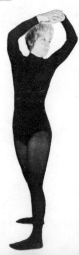

Standing Star—Step 3   *Standing Star—Step 4*

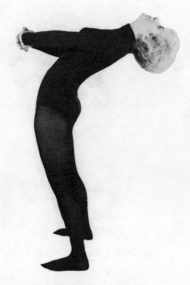

Standing Star—Step 5

Step 5: Extend the arms out in front of you, still palm to palm. Bend the body backward, and bounce the upper body backward to a count of five.

Beginning with Step 1, repeat each of the steps four times, then repeat the entire series three times, then twice, and finally once.

HAMSTRING STRETCHER

BENEFITS: Stretches and loosens the hamstring tendons, making the forward-bending postures easier

DIRECTIONS: Step 1: Lie flat on your back with arms at sides. Inhale, and bend the left knee.

Step 2: Straighten the knee until the toe is pointed toward the ceiling.

Step 3: Then, to get the maximum stretch for the hamstrings, try to point the heel toward the ceiling. Exhale as you lower the left leg to the floor; repeat with the right leg. Perform three times with each leg.

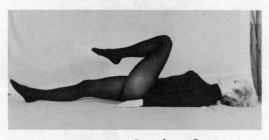

Hamstring Stretcher—Step 1

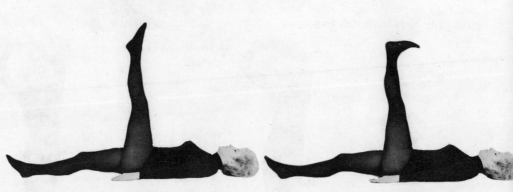

Hamstring Stretcher—Step 2   *Hamstring Stretcher—Step 3*

TWISTING POSE

BENEFITS: Eases many forms of backache • Removes stiffness from the spine

DIRECTIONS: Sit with legs outstretched in front of you; bend the right knee, and bring the heel up as close as possible to the buttocks. Now concentrate on your lower spine, and begin very slowly twisting the body to the right, starting at the lowest point of the spine. Continue twisting, visualizing each vertebra in turn twisting to the right. As you continue this twisting motion, bring both arms to the right side of your body, and place the palms flat on the floor so that, as you look down on them, the right outer hip is centered between the palms. Slowly turn the head as far as you can to the right. Remain in this position, breathing deeply and rhythmically, for thirty seconds. Repeat on the other side. Perform three twists in each direction. As you become more flexible, you may perform the Twisting Pose only once on each side, holding it up to two minutes.

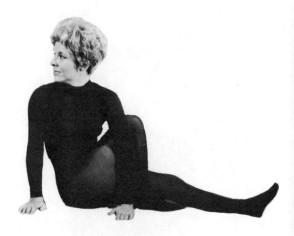

Twisting Pose

CROW

BENEFITS: Improves balance and concentration • Strengthens arms and wrists

DIRECTIONS: Squat on toes with hands on floor, a shoulder's width apart, spread fingers pointing forward. Place knees on upper arms, keeping lower arms straight. Then visualize the body as a large ball, and

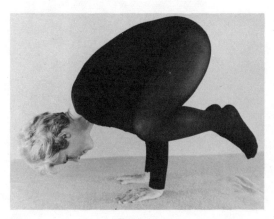

Crow

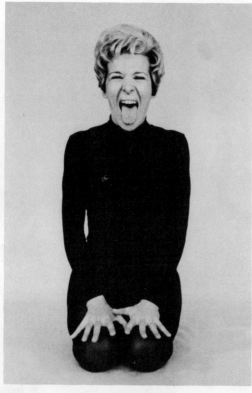

Lion

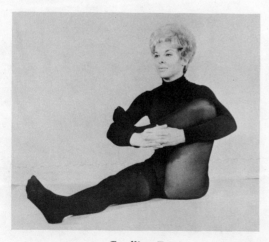

Cradling Foot

roll it up on the arms. The arms are bent at the elbows to give the knees a firm base. Lift toes off the floor, and try to balance, working up to thirty seconds.

LION

BENEFITS: Combats sore throat by sending an increased supply of blood into the throat and neck area • Tones the muscles and ligaments of the throat • Improves complexion • Helps eliminate double chin

DIRECTIONS: Sit with feet under you, sitting back on the heels. Place hands on knees as shown. Inhale deeply, and without exhaling stick the tongue out as far as possible, spread the fingers, and tense the entire body, particularly the neck and throat area. Maintain the tension of this posture for several seconds, then exhale and relax. Under normal conditions repeat the Lion two or three times. However, if you are on the verge of a sore throat, perform six to ten times, and repeat several times during the day. Adults find this posture somewhat embarrassing, but kids love it!

CRADLING FOOT

BENEFITS: Loosens thigh joints to facilitate the Lotus pose • Firms and slims the buttocks

DIRECTIONS: Pick the left foot up, and place in the bend of the right elbow. Interlock the fingers as shown so that the knee is cradled in the left elbow. Rock the cradled foot from side to side several times until the thigh feels loosened. Repeat with the other leg.

CRADLING FOOT— VARIATION

BENEFITS: Loosens tight hamstring tendons

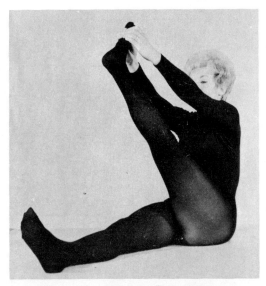

Cradling Foot—Variation

DIRECTIONS: After cradling each foot, grasp the·toes of the left foot, and pull them toward you as you extend the leg as shown. The more the toes are pulled down, the greater the stretch for the hamstrings.

ABDOMINAL LIFT

BENEFITS: Tones up all of the abdominal organs • Eliminates constipation • Reduces abdominal fat • Teaches control

PRECAUTIONS: Do not practice this series of exercises if you have an ulcer or a hiatal hernia, or if you are menstruating, pregnant, or have been fitted with an interuterine device for birth-control purposes. Perform this exercise in the morning when the bowels and bladder are empty and before you have eaten.

DIRECTIONS: Stand with feet slightly apart, hands on the fronts of the thighs, knees slightly bent, and

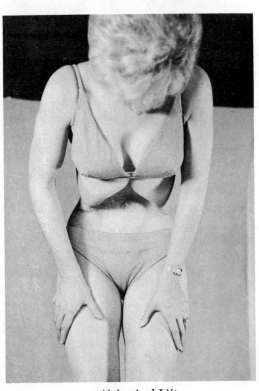

Abdominal Lift

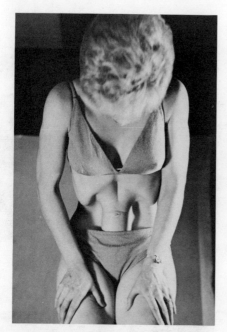

Uddiyana

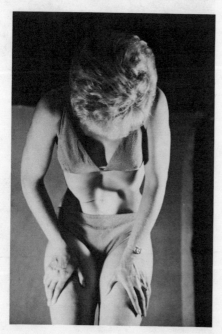

Nauli—Right Side

the chin pressed firmly into the chest. Inhale a complete breath through your nose, then exhale forcibly *through your mouth* until the lungs are completely empty. *Do not inhale again; hold the lungs empty.* Now pull the area above your navel back and up until a triangular hollow space is created under the rib cage. This should be a very pronounced cavity and is not the same as merely pulling in the stomach. Still without inhaling, push the hands against the thighs; this will isolate the rectus abdominus muscle as shown in the Uddiyana photograph. Release the hand pressure on the thighs, and you will again see the triangular hollow space in the Abdominal Lift photo. The object of this exercise is to execute the Abdominal Lift, then rhythmically press-release-press-release, which will create the abdominal muscles standing out, then being snapped back in. Do this as many times as you can without taking a breath. When you feel the need to breathe, remove the chin pressure, stand up, and relax for a minute or so, then repeat. Perform the exercise two or three times, and try to increase the numbers of in-and-out movements you can make. You should eventually be able to perform Uddiyana without pushing down with your hands—simply by using your mind.

NAULI

DIRECTIONS: After you have mastered Uddiyana, which is an in-and-out movement, you will be ready to try Nauli, which is a churning, wavelike sideways movement of the abdominal muscles. Perform the Abdominal Lift, then press down with the right hand on the right thigh, and you will note that the muscle stands out in the right side of your abdomen as shown below. Release the right hand and press with the left hand, and the muscle will stand out in the left side of your abdomen. By pushing alternately with the right hand and then the left, you will produce a continuous churning motion that moves sideways across the abdomen. When you become proficient at this, try reversing the movement, pushing down first with the left hand, then the right, so that the muscles are making the same movement but going in the opposite direction.

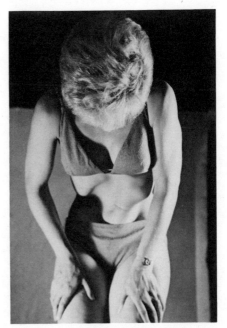

Nauli—Left Side

HAND AND WRIST EXERCISES

BENEFITS: Improves hands and wrists stiffened or sore due to arthritis, strain, or the aging process • Used as a preventive, it provides strong, flexible hands and wrists

DIRECTIONS: Step 1: Bend the elbows so hands are held in front of you, about six inches from the chest, palms facing each other with fingers pointed toward the ceiling.

Step 2: Clench the fists as tightly as possible, and hold for a count of ten.

Step 3: Now point the little finger toward the ceiling, using a firm, definite movement. Extend each finger in turn—the ring, middle, index fingers,

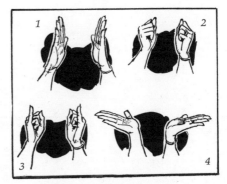

Hand and Wrist Exercises

and thumb—using brisk, precise movements until the fingers and thumb all point toward the ceiling.

Step 4: Bend the hands sharply at the wrists until the hands form 90° angles to the wrists, as shown. Now shake the hands ten times as though shaking off water. Repeat the sequence three times.

I can personally vouch for the dramatic effectiveness of this exercise. My right wrist had remained painful for three months following a sprain and was completely pain-free after performing this exercise daily for ten days.

FOOT EXERCISES

BENEFITS: Increases circulation in feet • These exercises are especially valuable for elderly people and for diabetics

DIRECTIONS: Step 1: Sit on floor or on a comfortable chair or sofa, and pick up the left foot in the left hand, resting the foot on your right knee. With right thumb and index finger firmly grasp the big toe of the left foot, and twist it to the right, then the left—repeating four times in each direction; then pull each toe a couple of times. Proceed to the next toe, repeating the above procedure until all five toes have been rotated four times each way, and pulled.

Step 2: Holding the left foot in left hand, grasp all the toes firmly in right hand with bottoms of toes in the palm of right hand. Firmly bend the toes up as far as they will go. Now place the tops of the toes in the palm of the right hand, and bend them as far down as they will go. Repeat four times in each direction, alternating up and down.

Step 3: Place left hand across the top of left foot, and squeeze until a groove appears on the sole of the foot. March the thumb of right hand down the groove four times.

Step 4: Place the palms of both hands at right angles to both sides of the left foot. With fingers together and outstretched, rapidly massage the sides of the foot by pulling the left hand toward you while pushing the right hand away from you. This motion is similar to rubbing the palms of the hands together except that the foot is between the palms.

Step 5: Grasp the left leg just above the ankle with the left hand, and grasp the toes with the right hand. Rotate the foot several times as if you were sharpening a pencil. Then go in the opposite direction. You will notice a tingling feeling in the entire foot and lower leg as the circulation is increased in this area. Repeat the entire series of exercises with the other foot.

CORPSE

BENEFITS: This is the recommended posture to assume for the complete relaxation period following the asanas, and also for resting between the various postures

DIRECTIONS: Lie flat on your

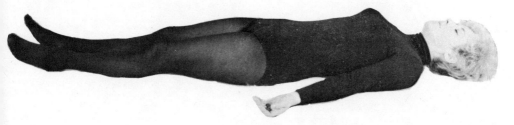

Corpse

back, arms relaxed at your sides, palms up. Allow the feet to turn slightly to the outside as the legs and ankles relax. During relaxation periods perform the complete yoga breathing described in Chapter 3.

CROCODILE

The Crocodile is a substitute for the Corpse that can be used for relaxation by those who are uncomfortable lying on their backs. This is particularly true of those with extreme swayback.

DIRECTIONS: Lie on the stomach with legs apart, toes turned in. Fold the arms so that the left hand lightly grasps the upper right arm and the right hand is placed in the same position on the left arm. Rest your forehead on your arms, and breathe deeply and rhythmically.

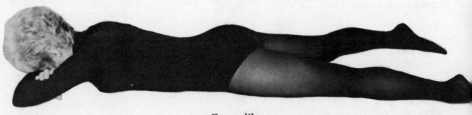

Crocodile

5

DIET AND NUTRITION

The yoga approach to food is in tune with the times. Pollution and ecology are becoming household words, and the yoga diet is highly unpolluted—ecology in its most personal form. Yoga is a way of life, and nutrition is part of that way. Accordingly, food plays a significant role in building a healthy body and mind.

In both ecology and nutrition man pays for breaking nature's laws. Whether these laws are broken intentionally or through lack of knowledge, the effects are in direct proportion to the breach. The average American male between the ages of forty and fifty is a good example of this cause-and-effect relationship. After years of improper eating and health habits, the body begins to protest, and the end results are heart attacks, ulcers, and other middle-age ills.

In fact, according to United Nations figures, a forty-year-old man in America has less chance of living to the age of fifty than men in fifteen other countries.

A purist yoga diet would be entirely vegetarian, but remember that yoga originated several thousand years ago in India. The climate is extremely hot, and there was no refrigeration. We have a temperate climate that makes meat, fish, and poultry more accessible, and we have refrigeration to slow down the spoilage rate. India's worship of the sacred cow was also a factor for not including meat in the diet.

A Look at Vegetarianism

The practice of living on a meatless diet is centuries old, but the term "vegetarianism" came into use only in the 1840s. This concept is attracting the attention of many young people today. Some American yoga teachers adhere strictly to a vegetarian diet; others do not insist upon it but stress a balanced diet of natural foods that are not overly processed or refined.

Although meat intake should be limited for many reasons, some books on vegetarianism state flatly that only vegetarians can expect to go to heaven. Consider the plight of the Eskimo—he must either emigrate or face forever the flaming inferno. I find it hard to believe that our Creator reserves the salvation of the soul exclusively for the inhabitants of the warmer climes.

One of the primary reasons for vegetarianism is reverence for life—the belief that man should not take the lives of animals to provide food.

Another vegetarian argument is that the teeth of living creatures are highly specialized and are an indication of the type of diet that best suits them. Horses and cows eat only plants and grain, and, as a matter of fact, they have short flat teeth well designed for their diet. Vegetarians argue that man's teeth resemble these, as contrasted to the long sharp teeth of lions, tigers, and the common house cat, which live primarily on meats that must be torn apart.

The beaver, whose large strong teeth grow continuously throughout life to replace areas that wear down due to constant use, supports the concept that Mother Nature knew the score when handing out teeth.

Geologist H. M. Ami reported in *Geography of North America* that the diet of prehistoric man did not include flesh in any form. Flesh-eating was unknown until the forests of nut trees and wild fruit trees were destroyed by the great ice cap that eroded the northern hemisphere during the glacial period.

The decision to eat meat or not is an individual one. However, if you're on the fence, syndicated medical columnist Dr. Lawrence Lamb points out that the incidence of atherosclerosis, a hardening of the arteries, is considerably less in vegetarians than that noted in meat-eaters.

Cleve Backster Shakes the Vegetarian World

Abstaining from meat to avoid taking life is an admirable sentiment, but recent research by Cleve Backster, a polygraph expert, shows that sentience, the capacity for feeling, extends much further than we had previously thought. People who accept the validity of only those facts of life that have withstood the test of time must be finding much of twentieth-century scientific research unnerving.

The notion that a plant has a complex emotional life, that it is capable of intense fear, sympathy, and perhaps the ability to read human minds is a bit far out for conventional thinkers. Or consider the fact that an egg "faints" just before it is broken and "gets nervous" when a neighboring egg is cracked. This sounds like just another science-fiction story, but it appeared in a page-one *Wall Street Journal* feature describing some of Mr. Backster's research on plants, eggs, fruits, and vegetables, and human blood and tissue samples.

Backster's research began in 1966 at the Backster School, where he teaches private investigators, police, and government personnel to use polygraph machines, better known as lie detectors. Wondering how long it would take water to travel from roots to leaves of a just-watered plant, he attached a polygraph electrode to a leaf and was amazed to note an immediate reaction similar to that of a person under emotional stimulation. Backster then decided to see if a plant would react in a similarly human manner if its safety were threatened. He decided to burn a leaf. Before he even reached for a match—in fact, at the moment the image of fire entered his mind—the plant registered extreme fear on the polygraph machine.

Backster's research on fruits and vegetables has been unsettling, to say the least, to many vegetarians. Three fresh vegetables were hooked up to polygraph electrodes, and one was selected to be dropped into boiling water. Before it was even touched, the selected vegetable victim fainted (this registers on the polygraph as a sudden upward bound, followed abruptly by a straight line).

In another experiment lots were drawn among six students to determine which one would uproot and tear to shreds one of two plants alone in a room. Later, the five guiltless students entered the room, and the remaining plant registered no reaction. When the plant-killer entered, the surviving plant fainted.

In another experiment an automated device selected tiny brine shrimp at random and dumped them into boiling water. Plants in another room that were hooked up to polygraph machines reacted at the instant the brine shrimp hit the water and died.

Backster's primary objective is to interest other scientists in conducting similar tests to see if they uphold his findings. Currently, he says, such research is being carried out in twenty-five or thirty universities. Aside from the added dimension his findings would contribute to scientific knowledge, he sees much deeper implications. Backster finds a definite correlation between his work and the power of prayer. He commented, "As a former agnostic who didn't take the trouble to be an atheist, I see some very high-level theological and spiritual implications of this. It opens the way for scientific exploration of the concept of the soul and seems to indicate a scientific justification for the power of prayer."

Similar experiments on plants have been performed, though not reinforced with electronic monitoring devices, and reported in Dr. Franklin Loehr's book, *The Power of Prayer on Plants*.

Should additional research prove, as Cleve Backster hints, that consciousness does, indeed, extend down to the single-cell level, it will require some serious rethinking about the cosmic scheme of things. I think it is safe to assume that the Creator would not place man on earth merely to starve or suffer the pangs of a guilty conscience. Just as smaller fish provide food for larger ones, and lesser animals are the primary diet of larger ones, this is obviously a necessary situation in maintaining a balance in nature.

The All-Important Protein

Vegetarians have markedly less heart disease, high blood pressure, and digestive and elimination disturbances than meat-eaters. Their main problem is in obtaining sufficient complete proteins in their diet. Proteins are the building blocks of the human organism and are required by every tissue in your body every day of your life. Proteins consist of amino acids, and there are twenty-two known amino acids, all of which are required for complete health. Of these twenty-two, eight are called essential amino acids, and a protein that contains all eight is called a complete or adequate protein. The remaining fourteen amino acids are also essential for health, but these can be manufactured by the cells from fat or sugar combined with the nitrogen freed from the breakdown of used proteins.

The best sources of complete proteins are meat, fish, fowl, eggs, fresh milk, powdered milk, buttermilk, yogurt, cheese, cottage cheese, soybeans, and powdered yeast. Among the complete proteins, some are better than others because they contain a greater supply of the essential amino acids. For example, egg yolk, fresh milk, liver, and kidneys are the most valuable complete proteins; roasts, steaks, and chops are complete proteins of lesser value because they contain smaller amounts of the essential amino acids. Generally, animal proteins—eggs, meat, fish, milk, and cheese—contain greater concentration of the essential eight amino acids than do the vegetable proteins.

Some sources of protein lack certain of the essential amino acids, but if they are eaten at the same meal as another protein that contains the missing elements, the proteins combine to make a complete protein. It is important that these be eaten at the same meal, however; should a missing element be eaten even one hour later, it is too late to form a complete protein.

Proteins form the foundation of good nutrition, and an extensive United States Department of Agriculture survey indicates that nine out of every ten Americans suffer from protein deficiencies. Another shocking paradox in our national nutritional situation is that even though 25 percent of Americans are seriously overweight, 10 percent of the population is anemic. Although anemia has many causes, a major one is protein deficiency.

Proteins are the most expensive of our essential nutrients, and the cost factor is a considerable one among low-income families. But faulty diets are the rule rather than the exception even among American families with high incomes. Many homemakers cater to the preferences of their families' palates, sacrificing good nutrition on the altar of supposedly good motherhood. Most of our widespread national malnutrition picture, though, is due to ignorance of the nutritional facts of life. The medical profession has provided scant assistance in the mass educational program that is needed, perhaps because doctors are restricted by time, and perhaps because they are more geared to treating ills than preventing them. The advertising of new food items, particularly snack items, compounds the problem by creating a demand for edibles of little nutritional value and diverting the food dollar into empty calories.

Protein Requirements

Even mothers who are concerned with good nutrition may be shortchanging their families unless they carefully plan their daily menus. Protein requirements, which are measured in grams, vary with age and sex. The Food and Nutrition Board of the National Research Council recommends the following amounts daily, although these figures, which must take into consideration the varying economic levels of our population, are generally considered by nutritionists to be too low.

Children under 12		*Children over 12*			*Adults*	
1–3	40 grams	Girls	13–15	80 grams	Men	70 grams
4–6	50 grams		16–20	75 grams	Women	60 grams
7–9	60 grams	Boys	13–15	85 grams	Pregnant	85 grams
10–12	70 grams		16–20	100 grams	Nursing	100 grams

Another way of arriving at the number of protein grams needed by adults is to divide each person's *ideal* weight by two. The result of this is approximately that person's daily protein gram requirement.

Listed below are some selected food items and their protein and caloric counts. These items are from the U.S. Department of Agriculture, *Agriculture Handbook No. 8* and *Home and Garden Bulletin No. 72.*

Food Item	Amount	Calories	Protein Grams
Cow's milk, whole	1 qt.	660	32
skim	1 qt.	360	36
Yogurt, of partially skim milk	1 cup	120	8
Cottage cheese, creamed	1 cup	240	30
uncreamed	1 cup	195	38
Cheese, American or cheddar	1 in. cube	70	4
Cheese, processed or Swiss	1 oz.	105	7
Eggs, boiled, poached, or raw	2	150	12
Eggs, scrambled or fried	2	220	13
Bacon, crisp, drained	2 slices	95	4
Beef, chuck, pot-roasted	3 oz.	245	23
Beef, commercial hamburger	3 oz.	245	21
Beef, lean ground	3 oz.	185	24
Beef, roast, oven-cooked	3 oz.	390	16
Beef, steak, as sirloin	3 oz.	330	20
Beef, steak, as round	3 oz.	220	24
Beef, dried or chipped	2 oz.	115	19
Chicken, broiled	3 oz.	185	23
Chicken, fried, breast or leg and thigh	3 oz.	245	25
Chicken livers, fried	3 medium	140	22
Lamb, chop, broiled (fat and lean)	4 oz.	480	24
Lamb, leg, roasted	3 oz.	314	20
Pork, chop	1 thick	260	16
Ham, pan-broiled	3 oz.	290	16
Turkey, roasted	3½ oz.	265	27
Liver, beef, sautéed with oil	3½ oz.	230	26
Liver, calves'	3½ oz.	261	29
Frankfurter, ¾" x 7"	2	246	14
Fish sticks, breaded, fried	5	200	19
Halibut, broiled	3½ oz.	182	26
Tuna, canned, drained	3 oz.	170	25
Beans, green, snap	1 cup	25	1
Beans, navy, baked with pork	¾ cup	250	11
Beans, red kidney, canned	1 cup	230	15
Bread, white	1 lb. loaf	1,225	39
Bread, whole wheat	1 lb. loaf	1,110	48
Cornflakes	1 cup	110	2
Oatmeal	1 cup	150	5
Rolls, breakfast	1 large	411	3
Shredded Wheat	1 biscuit	100	3

Food Item	Amount	Calories	Protein Grams
Wheat germ	1 cup	245	17
Almonds, dried	½ cup	435	13
Brazil nuts, unsalted	½ cup	457	10
Cashews, unsalted	½ cup	392	12
Peanut butter	⅓ cup	300	12
Sunflower seeds	½ cup	280	12
Brewers' yeast, powdered	½ cup	182	26

The Modern Approach to Diet

Mark Twain once remarked, "I never worry about what I eat. I just put the foods in my stomach and let them fight it out." This approach may have worked fine for Twain, but modern nutritionists and yoga devotees doubt it. They subscribe more to the theory that "you are what you eat."

The yoga approach to diet has a certain mystique and is surrounded by many legends, some of them erroneous. I once heard a yoga teacher announce in class that gaining weight is impossible for anyone regularly performing yoga postures. Don't believe it. Excess calories still produce excess weight.

Regular performance of yoga postures can, however, change your attitudes toward food. As your body shapes up, you treat it with more respect and prefer somewhat instinctively what your particular constitution requires. Much of yoga must be experienced to be believed, and the effect it has on one's attitude toward food is typical. Many students report a definite change in this area and a real preference for those foods that provide sound nutrition. Frequently, a student will develop a craving for specific foods, an indication that the body lacks an element contained in that food. This is an example of the body's intelligence in action. And as the body becomes better conditioned through yoga postures, it refuses to tolerate in the system any food that is toxic. A food that merely caused indigestion previously will now create allergy symptoms.

Yoga stresses each person's individuality and the innate wisdom and intelligence of the body. One of its objectives is to stimulate and awaken this wisdom and to trust it as a guide to eating habits. Yoga offers nutritional guidelines, but diet is a very individual thing. What foods are best for you depends on your physical condition, body type, height and weight, age, occupation, and way of life.

Inches off—Weight Stays the Same

A common occurrence in yoga classes, and a delightful one, is that many people find that measurements in inches decrease while the body weight remains constant. The person is actually smaller and slimmer, sometimes as much as two entire dress sizes, yet the weight registered on the scale remains unchanged. What is happening is a general restructuring of the organism, body fat being whittled away and firm muscular tissue replacing it. Many people are unaware that muscle weighs more than fat—in fact, about four times as much. No one has ever developed the unattractive bulging muscles associated with weight lifters through the practice of yoga. Rather, the yoga devotee can expect to be rewarded with a well-toned body. Because muscle tissue does weigh more than fat, a totally new figure can emerge from the old lumps and bulges without the scale ever being aware that anything is happening.

Individual Requirements

Everyone requires proteins, carbohydrates, fats, and vitamins and minerals. The ideal diet is provided by properly balancing these elements according to individual requirements. And these individual requirements keep changing throughout life.

For example, the growth years require more calories and a higher proportion of carbohydrates. From approximately twenty-five to forty-five, fewer calories and carbohydrates but more proteins are required. In later years a balanced diet should contain still fewer calories and fats while maintaining protein intake.

Nutrition experts warn that our eating habits are slowly but surely damaging the health of the entire nation. Government tests place our national physical fitness far below that of other countries. And man, of all the animals, is said to have the least knowledge in the proper management of his own body.

Mark Twain to the contrary, planning is the first step in the direction of proper eating. Experiment with natural foods, and determine which ones give you sufficient energy, proper weight, and a general feeling of well-being. Organize your findings into an eating plan, then stick to it.

Yoga is based on natural laws and stresses natural foods—those that are fresh, clean, pure, and unprocessed. Many of our dietary ills result from dependence on food that is overly processed—canned, preserved, pickled, bottled, bleached, polished, refined, and otherwise devitalized.

Just What Are Refined Foods?

Refined foods have been under constant attack in the medical and lay press, but exactly what are refined foods? Refined foods are those whose original state has been changed by processing, pickling, bleaching, the insertion of additives, and other alterations. Cakes and candy are good examples. Sugar, a refined product, contains almost nothing but carbohydrates without minerals, roughage, or vitamins. Food items made principally from refined sugar, syrups, and other concentrated sweets are refined foods.

Bread has been called the staff of life, but the reference by no means applies to the white bread so popular with many Americans which won't even keep a rat alive. Dr. Roger J. Williams, a University of Texas nutrition expert, experimentally fed sixty-four rats on nothing but so-called enriched bread, and within ninety days, forty had died of malnutrition. Those still alive were "severely stunted."

White bread is made of white flour that has had the husk and germ of the wheat removed. Even though it is enriched by vitamins so that it eventually has more vitamins than the original wheat, it has been stripped of its roughage qualities.

The United States has a higher incidence of colon disease than many other countries, and many experts blame our extensive use of refined foods. Refined foods lack bulk and roughage and lead to constipation, irritable colon, and colitis. On a world basis those countries that consume a great many refined foods have a higher incidence of cancer of the colon than countries favoring less refined diets that contain more roughage.

Empty Calories

Obesity is epidemic in America, and food processing is a contributing factor. Heavily processed food lacks vitamins, minerals, and basic nutrients, but still contains calories. Hence, the term "empty calories." Your body, lacking vital nutritional elements, craves and consumes more and more food.

The "empty calorie" label applies particularly to white bread, white sugar, white flour, and white rice, which have been refined until little food value remains. For better health, replace these with whole-grain breads and flour, brown rice, and raw sugar. And the best sweetener available is natural honey, unheated and unprocessed, available in health-food stores.

A medical survey of vitamin and mineral nutrition, covering the years 1950 through 1968, indicated that while the average American diet is generally nutritionally inadequate, *it got worse* in the decade between 1958 and 1968. During that same period there was a 65 percent increase in the consumption of sweet goods.

Sugar is a necessary element of nutrition; it is from the sugar and starch in carbohydrates that we obtain energy. However, nutritionists maintain that too much of the wrong kind of sugar is responsible for much of our self-inflicted malnutrition. Sugar brings to mind the white table variety found in most homes and in all restaurants. This is only one variety, called sucrose, and in its refined form is the most objectionable from a nutritional standpoint. Sucrose occurs naturally in many foods, and these are not to be avoided because they have not been refined.

Practically every food you eat contains natural sugar or potential sugar in one form or another. Fructose, or fruit sugar, is contained in all fruits. Glucose is the type of sugar in the blood, and lactose is the type of sugar found in milk.

Without ever touching a grain of refined table sugar, the healthy individual eating a varied diet will consume all the necessary carbohydrates needed for sufficient energy. When additional sweetening is needed, honey is preferred because glucose, the sugar found in honey, seems for some unknown reason to be less harmful than sucrose, or table sugar.

Much of the individual daily diet should be made up of fresh, raw foods such as fruits, vegetables, salads, and juices. Juices should be consumed within fifteen minutes after being prepared because they begin to lose their enzymes after that time. Fresh foods are always preferable, and frozen ones are next best. Canned foods lose a great deal of their nutritional value in the canning process.

American cooks could learn much from the French, particularly when it comes to cooking vegetables. Americans have a tendency to overcook fresh vegetables, which destroys much of their natural vitamin and mineral content. Those vegetables that are cooked should be considered done when they are crisp and tender, but not soggy. Very little water should be used, and that which remains should be served with the food.

Human Nutritional Requirements

There are forty known nutrients essential for optimum health that cannot be made in the body and must be obtained through food or vitamin supplements. These include fifteen vitamins, fourteen minerals, ten amino acids, and one essential fatty acid.

What's Wrong with the American Diet?

A justifiable criticism leveled at the American diet is that besides containing far too many refined foods and sweets, nearly all the proteins come from meat. And the preferred meats—steaks, roasts, and chops—contain less valuable sources of protein than the previously mentioned liver, kidney, yogurt, and other dairy products. The steak, baked potato, and salad diet so popular here makes vitamin and mineral deficiencies almost inevitable. Excess meat-eating is also thought to raise the uric-acid level in the body, a condition leading to the painful disease called gout.

Esoterically, ancient yoga treatises classify food in three categories: *sattvic* (pure), *rajasic* (stimulating), and *tamasic* (impure, overripe, or rotted). In the sattvic category are whole grains, milk, butter, fruits, and vegetables. The rajasic, or stimulating foods, include meat, fish, alcohol, coffee, and spicy foods that stimulate the nervous system. Tamasic foods are those that have started to decompose.

These treatises further state that man's food preferences are an indication of his mental and spiritual qualities. As man gradually becomes more mentally and spiritually advanced, his tastes in food become more pure. If this is true, America can look with pride to those young people who are shunning the steak and martini path in favor of natural and unrefined foods. Another ray of hope is that once people begin to include natural and pure foods in their diets, they rarely go back to stimulating or impure diets.

Another legitimate attack on our eating habits centers on the fact that we are a nation of gulpers, always so pressed by time or temperament that we do not chew our food thoroughly. It is well to remember that the stomach has no teeth and that chewing is the first step in digestion. Many nutrients cannot be assimilated unless food is well masticated. Insufficiently chewed food requires more digestive juices and acids to break down nutrients into usable components; this increased acidity contributes to such conditions as ulcers and gas. Washing each bite of food down with liquids also dilutes the necessary digestive juices and should be avoided.

The All-American Coffee Break

One of the few yogic disciplines that Indra Devi found burdensome during her training period was her Indian teacher's instruction to eliminate coffee and tea from her diet. Tea didn't appeal to her, but she really enjoyed coffee, as do most Americans.

Avoidance of stimulants is an age-old tenet of yoga, and current medical opinion substantiates yoga's belief that coffee is harmful to the human body. It is well known that ulcer patients must forgo coffee because it increases the amount and concentration of stomach acid.

Some of the other deleterious effects of coffee are less widely known, such as its relationship to heart disease. In our coffee-drinking nation heart disease accounts for 50 percent of all deaths—ten times higher than in most civilized countries. One medical study of two thousand men observed over a seven-year period showed that those who developed coronary disease drank five cups or more of coffee daily. Besides providing a morning pickup, even a single cup acts as a stress in the system and produces an immediate rise in blood fats and cholesterol.

The decaffeinated brands of coffee are much less harmful to the system. For those accustomed to the stimulus of caffein, an outright change to a decaffeinated brand would probably result in an unplanned midmorning snooze—or at least a pronounced letdown. Change the coffee habit gradually by brewing half regular and half decaffeinated coffee, and over a period of time increase the ratio of decaffeinated to regular until you are using primarily the low-caffeine variety.

Heavy coffee drinking also increases urine production and washes from the system the all-important B vitamins especially needed to offset stress. In fact, of the forty nutrients required for health, all but five—vitamins A, D, E, K, and linoleic acid—are readily lost in urine. Excess quantities of any liquid, including water, or the taking of diuretics also produce this effect.

And dieters who take the coffee route to weight loss may be compounding their problem. As potassium is washed from the system, sodium and water pass into the cells and result in fluid retention. Even though calorie intake is restricted, little weight loss is registered.

To enjoy good health, a proper balance must be maintained between the nutritional intake and the vitamin and mineral depletion caused by our biochemical individuality and way of life.

Safe Snacking

Americans are a nation of snackers. Unfortunately, most of what they snack on contributes nothing but nutritionless empty calories. Candy, colas, and sweets produce a quick energy surge, followed by a letdown as the pancreas secretes insulin, too much sugar resulting in an "overkill" reaction by the pancreas. When this additional insulin is secreted, energy goes down. The letdown after alcohol's initial pickup occurs for the same reason.

Tastes are cultivated, and they should be directed toward snacks that contribute toward the total nutritional picture. After all, every bite that you eat is reflected in your overall health picture. My children have lunch at school, and school lunch programs are notoriously low in protein. To make sure their after-school snack contains more than calories, I keep airtight containers of pumpkin seeds, sunflower seeds, sea-salted soybeans, raw nuts, and dried fruit on the counter they pass when entering the kitchen. Like most kids, they eat whatever's in sight, and these snacks provide nutrition and not just calories. I also keep a container of natural vitamin C (acerola and rose hips) on that counter because they can't take too much of this all-important vitamin. Their dentist maintains that the reason neither of these children has ever had a cavity is their daily intake of chewable vitamin C. If they are really hungry, they have a sandwich of whole-wheat bread and tuna fish, cheese, or dried beef, and milk, a snack that contains as much as twenty-four grams of protein, nearly half their minimum daily requirement. Though their tremendous energy and exuberance is often an affront to my yogic love of silence, they are, happily, very healthy.

Fasting—Pros and Cons

Fasting, the abstaining from all food, or at least from all solid food, is a controversial subject among yoga authorities. Those who fast do so for reasons such as discipline, increased spirituality, cleansing of the system, and weight control.

Those who oppose fasting contend that if a proper diet is followed, the system does not accumulate impurities and the fast is unnecessary. There are authorities backing both viewpoints, but the present state of environmental pollution is probably tipping the scales in favor of the fasters.

Fasting advocates recommend a twenty-four-hour fast each week. No solid food is taken, and intake is restricted to water and fruit and vegetable juices. Fresh juices are preferable to canned or frozen ones, because, as already stated, juices lose their enzymes soon after preparation. The fast can extend from noon of one day until noon of the following day, or any other convenient twenty-four-hour period.

On a twenty-four-hour water fast the average person loses 2 to 2½ pounds, and the regimen gives the digestive system a rest and increases the feeling of self-discipline and control. Heightened sensitivity or awareness is another favorable by-product.

How to Break the Fast

One of the advantages of fasting from one noon until the next is that no
full morning-to-night period passes with the stomach completely empty.
In eliminating food for a full day, one is actually fasting from the evening
meal of one day, throughout the day and the night of the next day, and
until arising on the third day. Abstaining from food for such an extended
period makes it imperative that the fast be broken carefully to avoid a
terrific stomachache.

Each person who fasts with regularity has a preferred method for breaking the fast, but the most important things to remember are not to eat too
much food at once, to avoid gulping, and to chew all food thoroughly.
Fresh fruits and freshly squeezed juices are good fast-breakers. My favorite is grated apples mixed with honey. Unbuttered whole-wheat toast with
oatmeal, honey, and milk is also acceptable. Be sure that the first food
is not oily or greasy. On one of my first fasts I returned to food with a
fresh vegetable salad—with an oil and vinegar dressing—and suffered for
my lack of wisdom for the remainder of the day.

The Importance of Acid-Alkaline Balance

Balance is vital in all phases of life, but perhaps it is most important in
the area of nutrition. All foods are either acid or alkaline in the system.
Some acid foods are necessary, but approximately 75 percent of all food
ingested should be alkaline. The body normally contains 75 percent alkaline elements and 25 percent acid. When this balance is consistently disturbed through improper eating habits, the entire system is eventually
weakened and becomes more susceptible to disease.

Meat, fish, poultry, coffee, tea, alcohol, fried foods, white flour, white
sugar, and white rice are all acid-forming to varying degrees. On the alkaline side, surprisingly, are lemons, grapefruit, oranges, and milk. Green,
leafy vegetables and most raw vegetables also are alkaline.

I am particularly conscious of the importance of the acid-alkaline balance because of an experience my mother had in the late 1950s. She had
suffered from rheumatoid arthritis for several years, had consulted medical
doctors with little success, and at that time was experiencing additional
problems due to the side effects of the cortisone medication she was
taking. She had written to the Mayo Clinic and was told, essentially, "Don't
come—there is nothing we can do to help you."

At this stage of her illness she was in constant severe pain and had great
difficulty using her hands or even walking. The next step obviously was a

wheelchair. In desperation she decided to visit the Ball Clinic (now the Mid-West Arthritis and Rheumatism Clinic), located in Excelsior Springs, Missouri. Because part of the treatment at that time involved osteopathic adjustment, the clinic was controversial in medical circles.

The first step in her treatment was total fasting and elimination of all medication. After that she was given buttermilk enemas to normalize intestinal bacteria, was placed on a specialized diet, and was given regular osteopathic adjustments.

Six weeks later she came home, a new person. All pain had disappeared as well as the difficulty in walking. Her disease, though incurable, had been arrested, and she was instructed to stay on the diet she had been given for the rest of her life. This diet, though not called a yoga diet, incorporates yogic beliefs in the selection of food.

I am reprinting below a table listing alkaline- and acid-producing foods followed by the clinic's dietary notes that she followed so successfully. Though I am not recommending that anyone treat his own illness, arthritis sufferers who have found little relief elsewhere may find this approach helpful. My mother has followed this diet, and her arthritis has remained in remission.

ALKALINE- AND ACID-PRODUCING FOODS IN THE HUMAN BODY

Acid-Producing Foods

All breads	Ham	Pies
All cereals	Hominy	Pork
Cakes	Hot cakes	Preserves
Coffee	Ice cream	Rice, polished
Cookies	Jams	Sausages
Cornmeal	Jellies	Soda crackers
Cornstarch	Lard	Spaghetti
Canned fish	Lean meats	Sugars
Eggs	Oatmeal	Syrups
Fat meats	Oleomargarine	Tapioca
Fish	Oysters	Tea
Fowl	Pastry	Alcoholic beverages

Alkaline-Producing Foods

Almonds	Brazil nuts	Cheese, cottage
Apples	Butter beans	Cheese, cream
Apricots	Cabbage	Cherries
Asparagus	Cantaloupe	Chestnuts
Bananas	Carrots	Coconuts
Beets	Cauliflower	Corn, canned
Blackberries	Celery	Cranberries

Alkaline-Producing Foods

Cucumbers	Lemons	Potatoes, Irish
Currants	Lettuce	Potatoes, sweet
Dates	Maple syrup	Prunes
Dried fruits	Milk	Radishes
Dried peas	Molasses	Raisins
Figs	Navy beans	Rhubarb
Filberts	Olives	Spinach
Grapes	Onions	Squash
Grapefruit	Oranges	Strawberries
Gooseberries	Parsnips	Tomatoes
Green beans	Peaches	Turnips
Green dandelion	Pears	Vegetable soup
Green peas	Pecans	Walnuts
Honey	Plums	Watermelon

Whole-grain foods are approximately neutral.

Note that the principal alkaline-producing foods include milk, nuts, and all kinds of green vegetables and ripe fruits. Almost all other foods are acid-producing in the body, including all kinds of breads, cereals, and other starch foods, all meats, fish, fowl, and eggs, all kinds of sugars, sweets, and pastry as well as pork, lard, and other animal fats.

SUGGESTIONS FOR HELPING TO PRODUCE AND MAINTAIN SYSTEMIC ALKALINITY AND CORRECT SYSTEMIC ACIDITY

1. Eat more milk, green vegetables, ripe fruits, and nuts and less of all other foods, and do not eat too much of any one kind of food.

2. Sugar, and products into which sugar enters largely, is the most acid-producing food known and should be limited or eliminated.

3. Next to sugar products, breads, cereals, and other starch foods are the most acid-producing and should be very markedly limited.

4. The next most acid-producing foods include all kinds of meats, fish, fowl, and eggs, all of which should be used very sparingly.

5. Bacon, lard, and other animal fats are acid-producing and must be used sparingly by all who are inclined to systemic acidity.

6. An abundance of whole milk is the best alkaline-producing food. One or two glasses should be taken three times daily with meals.

7. The next most alkaline-producing foods are oranges, lemons, grapefruit, tomatoes, all acid-tasting fruits, and all leafy vegetables.

8. Vegetables properly prepared are alkaline-producing, and those growing above the ground are most alkaline; vegetables should be used liberally.

9. All kinds of fruits, whether fresh, dried, or canned, are alkaline-producing unless too much sugar is used in their preparation.

10. Let morning meals be composed largely of fruits and milk; use no eggs, bacon, or meats and very little bread or breakfast foods.

11. Let the evening meal consist of a simple menu largely of alkaline-producing foods including milk and limited acid-producing foods.

The Fruit Fast

When digestive disturbances suggest that the acid-alkaline ratio is out of kilter, a fruit fast is a good way to regain balance. Two or three days of eating only fruits, preferably grown organically, is generally sufficient to cleanse the system of the residue of indiscreet food selection.

All animals, except man, voluntarily abstain from food when ill. When the organism is in the trauma of disease, the energy required to digest food slows down the healing process.

Vitamin Supplements

Public interest in the subject of vitamin supplements has risen along with the growing concern with ecology and what mishandling of our environment has done to the quality of food available to us. There are valid pro and con arguments on the vitamin issue. Many medical authorities maintain that vitamin supplements are unnecessary provided an adequate diet is eaten regularly. Those in favor of supplements counter that modern food growing, storage, and long-distance shipping strip much of the food value from food before it ever reaches the consumer, making it impossible to obtain an adequate diet.

Chemical fertilizers decrease the vitamin and mineral content in many foods, and storage decreases it more. In addition, canning, freezing, and cooking all take their toll, and unless food is thoroughly chewed, those nutrients that remain are not assimilated into the system. Even if everyone's diet were 100 percent adequate for his or her individual biochemical needs, consider these alarming facts: Stress robs the system of the B vitamins; vitamin C, which cannot be stored in the system, is destroyed by infections, many medications, smoke, smog, or smoking, pesticides, and the chemicals used in water purifiers; oral contraceptives increase the need for folic acid; diuretics induce potassium deficiencies; and drinking alcohol increases the requirements for B-complex vitamins and causes a high loss of magnesium through excessive urination.

These are just a few samples of how one's life-style affects those nutrients present in the system. There are many more comparable examples, and to render the situation even more confusing, no two people have exactly the same nutritional requirements. Also, since some vitamins and minerals require adequate supplies of other nutrients in the system in order to be utilized, it is almost impossible to have a single nutritional deficiency.

Should you feel that vitamin supplements might improve your general health, be prepared for a shock, followed by a feeling of intimidation or at least inadequacy, when you approach the vitamin counter of your drugstore or go into a health-food store. Vitamins can be either natural or synthetic, and there is a wide range of potency measured in terms called grams, micrograms, milligrams, and international units.

Natural vitamins are often thought superior to the synthetic ones, but they are frequently more expensive; chemically, the synthetic vitamin C and all B vitamins are identical to the natural ones. It is also difficult to take a sufficient quantity from a natural source, such as the massive doses of vitamin C recommended by many doctors for combating the common cold. Many authorities suggest that you take natural vitamins when possible, but be willing to accept the synthetic ones if necessary.

This is really a never-never land for the uninitiated. Minimum daily requirements of vitamins vary between the sexes and also in age groups, and for some nutrients the minimum daily requirement has not been established. Some vitamin pills are actually combinations of vitamins, and the proportion of each may vary from one brand of pills to another. The B-complex vitamins, which actually contain individual nutrients, are synergistic, which means that they must be present in specific proportions to be effective. In many B-complex formulas these proportions are not followed, even by reputable companies.

The use of vitamin supplements is one area where a little learning really is a dangerous thing. Should you decide to go into supplements, be prepared to spend considerable time learning what the requirements are for your age and sex, analyzing your diet to determine approximately which nutrients you may lack, and wading through the maze of milligrams and international units.

Calories and Life-Styles—Then and Now

At the turn of the century men consumed approximately 6,000 to 6,500 calories daily and women some 4,000 to 4,500. Today's averages are 2,400 to 2,800 for men and 1,800 to 2,200 for women, according to nutritionist Adelle Davis. And of today's daily calories, some two-thirds come from foods that have been refined to the extent that some or all of the nutrients have been discarded.

The main reason our grandparents could put away all those calories without incurring the obesity that plagues us today is largely because of exercise. We lead such sedentary lives compared to theirs that following their diet would produce a nation of human blimps.

Even though we eat less, heart specialist Paul Dudley White stated at an Oregon Heart Association meeting in July, 1972, that as a nation we are overfed and underexercised. He stated that our life-style is at the emergency stage and cites hardening of the arteries in children as young as two years old as an example. He strongly criticized American parents for driving their children to school and elsewhere instead of allowing them to walk, and said: "We must completely change our children's way of life. It's perfectly ridiculous the way they live."

Dr. White, then eighty-six, advocated vitamins, walking, bicycling, and climbing stairs instead of taking elevators. According to this expert, the American family must change its dietary habits and exercise regularly— and we can't wait another generation to begin!

6

STRESS AND TENSION

Prior to their first class, I have all my students fill out a physical information form, which asks for specifics regarding any serious illnesses or surgical operations they have had in the past two years; any medication they are taking and the purpose for which it was prescribed; any physical handicap or chronic condition that might affect their participation in a yoga class; and their blood-pressure reading, if it is higher than 150 or lower than 100. The last question on this form is "What do you hope to gain from the practice of yoga?"

Information on the physical condition of my students is extremely important to me because some students simply must not do some postures. But it is of equal importance to know what motivates these people to seek out a yoga class. Many of them come because it is the "in" way to physical fitness and because it does produce dramatic shape-up results. Some are drawn by the spiritual and mystical aspects of the subject. But by far the majority come because they view it as their last hope in learning to relax and to cope with the tremendous pressures and stresses of the twentieth century.

All of us feel the effects of stress and tension, and yet few know anything really specific about stress. This chapter is devoted to explaining what stress is and how it affects you. Yoga helps combat stress in several ways, both physically and mentally. The postures themselves are beneficial in fighting stress because stretching releases the tension that builds up in muscles. And the complete relaxation that concludes each class doesn't just end there. Once students know the feeling of being completely relaxed, they can produce this physical state by recalling the feeling and mentally recreating it when they feel tension building up. Another way in which yoga aids in the fight against stress is by increasing awareness of what is going on inside you. Yoga gets you in touch with yourself, and this increased awareness allows you to ease the grip of tension.

Stress and tension are common words, and they are often erroneously thought to mean the same thing. Stress is frequently considered a universal enemy in our bustling lives, but actually we couldn't function at all without some stress. Lacking stress, we wouldn't even get out of bed in the morning or participate in life in any way. Too much stress, on the other hand, *is* the enemy—and it's a powerful one. Tension is one result, or symptom, of too much stress.

Modern science is indebted to Dr. Hans Selye, author of *The Stress of Life*, who is regarded as the world's foremost authority on stress. His research has provided what he calls a biological portrait of stress, or how stress actually affects the body. According to Dr. Selye, "Many people think of stress as nervous tension or some other thing. That is not true. Scientifically speaking, stress is a non-specific response of the body to any demand made upon it." The happy events in life can produce as much stress as the unhappy ones; watching your hometown team win the Super Bowl can be just as stressful, biochemically, as engaging in a violent argument with your mother-in-law.

No one can or should totally avoid stress, but too much of it can kill you. The adrenal glands, one perched atop each kidney, are your artillery to cope with the stress of life. Some twenty-eight hormones, including adrenaline, are secreted by the adrenals. These coordinate with other functions of the body in a highly integrated fashion. As long as stress is continued, the adrenals keep pouring their hormones into your system.

What Chronic Stress Does to You

Dr. Selye has discovered that you, the human being, go through three stages when subjected to chronic, continual stress. In the initial stage of stress you react with alarm. The physiological effects of the alarm stage, regardless of what causes the stress, are elevation of blood pressure and blood sugar, increase in stomach acid, and tightening of the arteries.

The second stage is a period of adjustment to the stress, during which calming hormones are secreted from the pituitary and the adrenals. In the third stage your defenses are exhausted, and the body breaks down. Everyone has a different breaking point; some individuals may break early in the stress game, and some may cope with it for a long time.

But with constant, unrelieved stress, the breakdown will come. Many diseases have been linked to stress—heart attacks, diabetes, migraine head-aches, and back problems are a few of them. Stress alone does not cause these diseases, but stress so debilitates the body that it breaks down at its weakest point. Those who are genetically predisposed to heart disorders will probably react to stress by having heart attacks. Those whose spines are their weakest link are candidates for a host of back problems.

Prehistoric man had two basic reactions to the stresses that beset him— fight or flight; he either fought the enemy or ran away. In either case his body was ready for it, the entire organism reacting to the adrenal hor-mones that flooded through his system.

Physical Reactions to Stress

These adrenal hormones cause the heart to race, the digestive processes to halt, the muscles to tense, the arteries to contract to prevent bleeding, and the blood chemistry to change so that if a wound is incurred, bleeding will be slower.

Civilization has polished the rough edges from our instinctive behav-ior. We no longer fight or run away, although our physical reaction pre-pares us for this response, and our bodies suffer because we don't. Instead of following our basic instincts, which haven't really changed much over the centuries, we take refuge in more socially acceptable behavior; we get ulcers, develop psychosomatic ills of all kinds, and are generally a nation suffering from the effects of too much unrelieved stress. This life-style, which is in tremendous conflict with our basic nature, is the result of cul-tural or social programming. Society expects us to act in certain ways, we have been conditioned to accept as proper this form of behavior, and so we perform according to the dictates of that programming.

Life Changes as Stressors

Nothing is constant except change, but too many changes occurring too quickly create the degree of stress that produces illness. The medical pro-fession has long known that many diseases are emotionally induced. In fact, Dr. John Schindler, in *How to Live 365 Days a Year*, suggests that 50 percent of all illness is emotionally induced. Dr. Andrew Weil, in *The Natural Mind*, goes further by stating that he believes *all* disease is psycho-somatic. But only recently has there been a listing of the various changes people encounter in life, with each change assigned a numerical designation indicating its potential for making you ill.

This listing, in chart form, appeared in the *Journal of Psychosomatic Research*, 1967, and is the result of two decades of research by Dr. Thomas H. Holmes, professor of psychiatry at the University of Washington School of Medicine in Seattle, and his colleague, Dr. Richard Rahe. The chart lists forty-three specific events that produce what they call "life crisis units." All the events listed require some degree of coping or adaptation.

Twentieth-century American life is undergoing changes at an unprecedented rate—changes in value systems, marital relationships, parent-child relationships, and just about everything else. These scientists, studying man's ability to adapt to change, have discovered that excess change—good or bad—will make eight out of ten persons ill.

Everyone knows that sorrow and disaster will often lead to illness; it is surprising, however, that achievement and happiness that produce change can also lead to illness. Of those people who score 300 or more life crisis units, 80 percent will become ill within a two-year period, although there is no way to tell which eight out of ten will be stricken. In yoga it is known that physical flexibility provides mental flexibility and stability as well. Perhaps this inner resilience is a key factor in coping with rampant change. Keep this in mind when totaling your life crisis units for the past two years.

To use this chart, add up the total life crisis units for the life events you have experienced in a given two-year period. The key to scoring your life crisis units is listed below:

0–150	No significant problems
150–199	Mild life crisis (33 percent chance of illness)
200–299	Moderate life crisis (50 percent chance of illness)
300 or over	Major life crisis (80 percent chance of illness)

SOCIAL READJUSTMENT RATING SCALE

Rank	Life Event	Life Crisis Units
1	Death of spouse	100
2	Divorce	73
3	Marital separation	65
4	Jail term	63
5	Death of close family member	63
6	Personal injury or illness	53
7	Marriage	50
8	Fired at work	47

Rank	Life Event	Life Crisis Units
9	Marital reconciliation	45
10	Retirement	45
11	Change in health of family member	44
12	Pregnancy	40
13	Sex difficulties	39
14	Gain of new family member	39
15	Business readjustment	39
16	Change in financial state	38
17	Death of a close friend	37
18	Change to different line of work	36
19	Change in number of arguments with spouse	35
20	Mortgage over $10,000	31
21	Foreclosure of mortgage or loan	30
22	Change in responsibilities at work	29
23	Son or daughter leaving home	29
24	Trouble with in-laws	29
25	Outstanding personal achievement	28
26	Wife begins or stops work	26
27	Begin or end school	26
28	Change in living conditions	25
29	Revision of personal habits	24
30	Trouble with boss	23
31	Change in work hours or conditions	20
32	Change in residence	20
33	Change in school	20
34	Change in recreation	19
35	Change in church activities	19
36	Change in social activities	18
37	Mortgage or loan less than $10,000	17
38	Change in sleeping habits	16
39	Change in number of family get-togethers	15
40	Change in eating habits	15
41	Vacation	13
42	Christmas	12
43	Minor violations of the law	11

The types of ailments and accidents suffered by those in Dr. Holmes's survey who became ill comprised a wide variety of psychiatric, medical, and surgical diseases, including cancer. Serious infections, allergic reactions, peptic ulcers, and headaches were frequently mentioned, as were colitis, high blood pressure, pains of joints or muscles, and nervous diarrhea.

According to an item in the May 29, 1972, issue of *Time* magazine, reprinted below with their permission, so-called unwanted pregnancies, though technically not an illness, may be another end result of too many life crises in too short a time span.

"Unwanted pregnancy" is a widely accepted term among both laymen and behavioral scientists. It is also widely misunderstood, according to Cornell University Psychiatrist Lawrence Downs and Psychologist David Clayson. In a paper presented to the American College of Obstetricians and Gynecologists, Downs and Clayson offer convincing evidence that among women who have abortions, pregnancy is initially "more wanted than unwanted." Far from being accidental, it represents a subconscious effort to cope with extreme emotional stress.

Downs and Clayson reached their conclusions after studying 108 patients at New York Hospital. Most of the women were well informed about birth control, and many had sometimes practiced it at some time in their lives. Then why, the investigators wondered, did such women get pregnant?

The answer seems to lie partly in the women's personalities, which proved to be quite different from those of a comparison group of 49 women hospitalized for the birth of their first or second babies. All of the women in the comparison group tested normal on the Minnesota Multiphasic Personality Inventory, a much-used measure of emotional health. By contrast, only 21 percent of the abortion patients were diagnosed as "normal"; 24 percent were revealed to be psychotic, and 55 percent were found to have neuroses or related disorders. In fact, more than a third of the abortion patients had sought professional help for their psychiatric problems in the year before they became pregnant.

Besides these inner difficulties, many of the abortion patients had suffered personal losses in the year or two prior to conception. In 47 percent of the cases, a member of the immediate family had died or been diagnosed as fatally ill. The end of a marriage or of a longstanding love relationship had been experienced by 43 percent. Some two-thirds of the abortion patients had sustained either or both of these losses, and a striking 85 percent of the abortion group had suffered either a personal loss or grave psychiatric disturbance, or both, in the months just before conception.

These percentages are the first statistical evidence that most abortion patients have conceived while under exceptional emotional stress. The results seem to support the widely accepted psychiatric belief that pregnancy is seldom a chance occurrence. Thus, Downs and Clayson conclude, the women they studied had unconsciously "chosen" pregnancy as a way of repairing "a threatened or damaged psyche." They needed their supposedly unwanted pregnancies, at least for a while, "to prove something to themselves"—perhaps that they were truly feminine, or that they were whole enough to create, or that they need not be entirely alone.

Physical Stress and Mental Stress

There are basically two kinds of stress—physical and mental—and the human body fights both in exactly the same way. Most people recognize some forms of stress easily but fail to realize that many accepted facets of everyday life are actually stressors.

A few of the overlooked stressors include noise, air pollution, cigarette smoking, alcohol, coffee, drugs and medication, boredom, infections, lack of sleep, an inadequate diet, vitamin deficiencies, and one's emotions. Of all the stressors, Dr. Selye contends that the three worst ones are emotions: hatred, frustration, and anxiety.

Frustration and anxiety have been produced in laboratory animals by forcibly restraining a normally active rat and placing a mouse in a cage next to a cat. Both the frustrated rat and the anxiety-ridden mouse reacted alike—they were literally stressed to death. No one can love everybody, but allowing yourself to hate, and to dwell on that hatred, is a most self-destructive emotion. Hatred's intensity is an inner-directed thing; it creates great stress and harms no one but the hater, who lays himself open to ulcers, high blood pressure, and heart disease. The mind-control aspect of yoga is extremely helpful in directing the concentration away from harmful and dangerous thinking.

The Stress in Your Life

An understanding of stress and what it can do to you is the first step in combating this potential killer. One of the physiological reactions to stress is an increase in stomach acids, and one of our primary stress diseases is the peptic ulcer. Perforated ulcers kill more than ten thousand Americans each year. In fact, one out of every ten of our citizens will get one or more ulcers sometime during his life, and it is estimated that more than ten million Americans now suffer from ulcers. Stress was long ago incriminated as a causative factor in ulcers, but Dr. Jay M. Weiss, a psychologist at Rockefeller University in New York City, has conducted experiments that pinpoint which types of stressors are most damaging—physical or psychological.

In physical stress experiments Dr. Weiss subjected an animal to an audible tone that was followed ten seconds later by an electric shock. The animal learned that it could prevent the shock by jumping to a platform. To test for psychological stress, a second animal was wired to the first; it also heard the tone, but nothing the second animal did could prevent the shock. If the first animal didn't jump fast enough, the second one received a shock. In this test the second animal developed many more ulcers than the first, proving that being helpless to control its circumstances was far more damaging than the electric shock that resulted. For the first time, Dr. Weiss proved that psychological stress is much deadlier than physical stress.

In the human realm people who face worries and problems try to cope with them and find solutions. If the solutions attempted *do* solve the problems, the risk of ulcers is minimal. But if a person tries repeatedly to solve the problems and no workable solution is found, he becomes a prime candidate for an ulcer. Dr. Weiss feels that the most important consideration in this theory is relevant feedback; when the stressed individual gets feedback that he is doing the right thing to solve the problem, the ulcer risk diminishes.

An example of the type of coping behavior that lessens ulcer risk is the businessman who has a personality conflict with his immediate superior. If the businessman tries to alleviate the conflict and finds that the relationship is improving, he runs little risk of developing an ulcer. On the other hand, if his efforts to ease the abrasiveness between them have no effect regardless of how hard he tries, he is in danger of getting an ulcer. When the stressed person is not in control of how his life is going, he provides an ideal situation for ulcer development.

Backache

As life becomes more stressful and hectic, the incidence of back problems goes up and up. The National Center for Health surveys indicate that more than 7 million Americans are being treated for chronic back pain, and 1.5 to 2 million new cases are added each year. Many doctors rate back pain as the second most common reason adults consult a doctor. (The primary cause for visits to a doctor is to seek treatment for respiratory complaints.)

Diagnosing the cause of back problems is complicated by the fact that many difficulties result from malfunctioning organs such as the kidneys, bladder, prostate, and even the stomach that manifest as lower-back pain. And spinal curvature (scoliosis) victims, many of whom are unaware of their abnormality, run sixty times the risk of developing back and neck problems compared to those whose spines are straight. Only a back specialist can be sure if you have spinal curvature. However, here are some things you can check yourself if you suffer from chronic back pain that defies diagnosis and treatment:

Stand in front of a full-length mirror without clothes, and check to see if (1) your shoulders are uneven, (2) one side of your chest protrudes beyond the other, or (3) your pelvis tilts a bit. See a back specialist if one or more of these irregularities exist.

Back victims often complain that they bent over to tie a shoelace and were stricken with sudden, debilitating back pain that gave no prior warning of anything being amiss. Although the symptoms may have come on abruptly, experts agree that usually the basic cause has been building for a long time, unless the pain stems from a fall, an automobile accident, lifting something heavy, or is induced by some other quick, unnatural movement. These authorities concur in blaming the victim's basic lifestyle; the event that triggered the acute pain was merely the straw that broke the camel's back, if you'll pardon the cliché.

Medical men are profile-prone these days, and they have a typical composite personality that is likely to develop a number of ills from heart disease to cancer. Their profile of the back victim is an office worker in the late thirties or forties, one who was physically active in high school and college but no longer gets any regular exercise, someone who is twenty or thirty pounds overweight with a high-pressure job that bothers him. People with sedentary jobs are high-risk candidates, because sitting places greater pressure on the disks in the lower lumbar region than standing.

The proverbial paunch is a common badge of the office worker and one that contributes greatly to lower-back pain. When the abdomen sags forward, it places great stress on the lumbar region, as any very pregnant woman will testify. Much low-back therapy consists of exercises to strengthen the abdominal muscles and diet to eliminate the midsection overhang. Regular practice of yoga asanas assures strong abdominal muscles, and many of the postures such as the Arch and its variations, leg-raising, rocking, and others are identical to exercises prescribed for faulty lower backs.

Dr. Hans Kraus, a specialist who treated President John F. Kennedy, wrote in *Backache, Stress, and Tension* that one out of every two Americans is underexercised. He states, "Under exercise is a major factor in causing back pain and tension syndrome (stiff neck and headache), and even emotional instability, duodenal ulcers, diabetes and heart disease."

Since stress strikes at one's weakest point, many people will react to it by developing backache at any place along the spine. Stress creates muscle tension, and this uptightness may well pull a vertebra out of alignment if nothing is done to release the accumulated tension. The twisting poses, Sitting Five-Step, Shoulder Pulls, the Cat Stretch, and neck exercises ease tension in specific areas, and general yoga practice eases tension throughout the body, helping many back sufferers.

Although the specialists don't agree on proportions, they do concur in stating that many of the back ills they treat are psychosomatic, or emotionally induced. Many feel that nearly all back problems have mental origins, because muscles tend to contract involuntarily when there is painful conflict or emotion. Nearly all of these experts agree that the way a person copes with the stresses of our modern civilization figures prominently in one's susceptibility to back ailments.

Pain in the Neck?

When was the last time someone gave you a pain in the neck? Though this phrase is usually said in jest, people and situations that annoy or irritate you, and the tension produced by these irritations, can be painful. Pain in the neck is emotionally induced in seventy-five out of one hundred patients with this complaint, according to Dr. John Schindler.

Each time someone or something irritates you, the shoulders raise and tighten a bit, and the muscles become tense. Minor annoyances occur many times each day, and unless something is done to work off the accompanying tension, painfully tight muscles will be the end result.

Tense muscles produce many of our general aches and pains, and the muscles that react most quickly to emotionally trying situations are those that are used most. The muscles at the back of the neck are frequently tight and tense because they are used more than any other set of skeletal muscles.

To check the tension level in your own neck area, let your head drop to your chest, then slowly roll it around to the right, keeping the shoulders still and letting the weight of the head carry itself around to the back, left, and returning to the original position. In one continuous slow movement roll the head four times to the right and then four times to the left. If these neck rolls make you feel drowsy, it indicates that much tension has built up, and the releasing of this tension produces the feeling of drowsiness. The neck exercises and the neck roll keep the neck tension-free.

Migraine Headache

Migraine headache has plagued mankind and the medical profession since ancient times. Its cause and cure still remain a mystery. Many doctors believe the causes of migraine headaches are psychosomatic, but regardless of the cause, they create great suffering for many people.

Stress is another suspected culprit. If so, it is an old enemy. Scientists have found skulls of prehistoric people with holes bored in them. These holes were ground through the bone with stone implements to allow the "evil spirits" to escape.

The Menninger Clinic in Topeka, Kansas, recently announced the results of some interesting experiments with migraine sufferers, which involve the use of the mind. During an attack of migraine headache it was discovered that the head of the sufferer was hot and the hands were cold.

The sufferers were taught to "think" their hands warm. When they succeeded in doing this, the headache disappeared. The warming of the hands could not be accomplished mechanically, as by placing them in warm water, but had to be channeled through the brain to be effective.

Many sufferers of common headache, and some migraine sufferers, find that their ailments disappear with the regular practice of yoga. The reason is simply that yoga lessens tension and works toward creating a generally healthier body tone.

Heart Disease and High Blood Pressure

Though heart disease doesn't possess quite the terror potential of cancer, it is the number-one killer in the United States. Some 600,000-plus Americans die from it each year; for more than half these people, their first heart attack struck without warning and was their last. Four out of ten heart-attack victims die before reaching the hospital. Dr. Paul Dudley White called heart and circulatory disease "an epidemic that endangers not only the aged but our young and middle-aged, from teen-agers up." In the thirty-five-to-forty-four age group, 30 percent of all deaths are from cardiovascular failures, and by age seventy-five, 70 percent of all deaths are due to heart disease.

Women suffer fewer heart attacks than men until menopause, then—particularly those hard-driving, time-pressured women who eat, smoke, or drink too much—find their chances of suffering a heart attack markedly increased. Meanwhile, high blood pressure, or hypertension, kills nearly as many females as males, regardless of age.

The U.S. Government's National Institutes of Health has begun a major campaign to reduce our heart-death toll. Their primary goal is to find out how to prevent arteriosclerosis, or hardening of the arteries, which has been linked with high cholesterol levels (a fatty substance in the blood-stream), high blood pressure, and heavy cigarette smoking.

Stress hits one's weakest area, and approximately 1 percent of our national population has an inherited high cholesterol level, a genetic irregularity that shortens their average life expectancy by twenty-five years. Obviously, controlling, coping with, and avoiding undue stress is imperative for these people, who account for between 30 and 50 percent of the 160,000 to 180,000 patients under fifty who die of heart attacks each year. While genetic inheritance is beyond our control, those afflicted with this disorder might profitably consider the fact that vegetarians have less incidence of arteriosclerosis than meat-eaters. And since cigarette smoking in itself is a stressor, it is hard to imagine anyone with this genetic time bomb even considering it.

Regular exercise is universally acclaimed as preventive therapy for heart disease, and although exercise alone doesn't eliminate stress, it does relieve the muscular tension created by stress. Unless tremendous changes are adopted, one out of every two Americans will eventually die of heart disease, our deadliest stress-related killer. This should motivate at least a few people to join exercise with proper diet, a positive mental attitude, and a life-style dedicated to one's own personal ecology program.

Hypertension, more commonly known as high blood pressure, is an affliction of approximately 22 million Americans. Ten percent of high blood pressure sufferers have what is called secondary hypertension, a type that is the result of a specific disease or physical abnormality. Fortunately, cures can be accomplished by means of medicine or surgery.

The remaining 90 percent suffer from essential hypertension, a hereditary problem for which the cause and cure are presently unknown, though some medical authorities believe it stems from an inherited malfunction of the kidneys or adrenal glands, complicated by psychological factors. Its treatment involves weight loss if the patient is overweight, and the prescription of antihypertension drugs.

Although Veterans Administration studies prove that lowering extremely high blood pressure reduces the incidence of strokes, kidney failure, and congestive heart failure, many experts are concerned about the long-term complications involved in taking potent blood-pressure-lowering pills.

An adjunct to the treatment of high blood pressure is to eliminate or drastically reduce the amount of sodium, or salt, in the diet. Salt helps retain water in body tissues and thus aggravates hypertension. Diuretics are frequently dispensed to eliminate some of the fluid accumulation. However, along with the excess fluid many vitamins and minerals are also lost. The continued use of diuretics can cause serious vitamin and mineral deficiencies, opening a veritable Pandora's box of ailments related to these deficiencies.

Those who suffer from high blood pressure can help themselves by becoming familiar with the sodium content of various foods and exerting the necessary discipline to remain on a low-salt diet. Japan has one of the highest hypertension death rates in the world, and their sodium intake is correspondingly high—14 grams per day in the southern islands and 26 grams per day in the north. The highly hypertensive American sodium intake is approximately 10 to 15 grams per day. Compare this to the Alaskan Eskimo's 1.6 grams per day and his very low incidence of high blood pressure.

Fluid retention, which also causes irritability, can be minimized by avoiding such high-sodium foods as dill pickles, sauerkraut, celery, ham, potato chips, and hot dogs, and by learning the sodium content of the foods normally eaten. All canned vegetables have added salt, and all meats and vegetables contain some sodium in their natural form.

Alcoholism

In discussing the drug problem in *The Natural Mind* Dr. Andrew Weil states his belief that man craves the experience of altered states of consciousness. He may well be right, because alcohol, a legal mind-altering drug, has been around since the Stone Age. It is the oldest drug known to man, and nearly every culture in the world, with the exception of the Eskimo, has developed some form of alcoholic beverage as a tension easer and an antidote for stress. And although alcohol is used presumably to offset the effects of stress, the way it acts in the human body makes it one of our most lethal stressors, and alcoholism our most serious stress-related disease.

Going into the physiological facts of alcohol may seem to be going rather far afield in a book devoted primarily to yoga, but it is actually highly pertinent. Many of the facts about how alcohol affects the human body are only now becoming known. Most people have viewed the consumption of alcoholic beverages primarily as a morning-after problem and not as a contributor to long-range problems. We are now discovering that the damage that can be caused is cumulative and doesn't end when the hangover abates.

While learning to relax through yoga provides a stress-relieving alternative to alcohol, its most important contribution is to increase the regard we have for our bodies. Yoga views the body as the living temple of the spirit and serious participants are disinclined to abuse that body.

Despite alcohol's long tenure as man's comfort and solace, the seriousness of the problems created by it have been largely overlooked until recently. Perhaps one good result, at least, has emerged from the marijuana and drug scene of the past decade: The counterclaim of drug advocates that their vice is less serious than the older generation's use of alcohol has stimulated society finally to take a hard look at the alcohol picture. The recently formed National Institute on Alcohol Abuse and Alcoholism, headed by Dr. Morris E. Chafetz, reports that alcoholism has become the nation's biggest untreated disease and that alcohol is the nation's most abused drug. Many of the institute's findings reported to Congress are shockers.

The general impression held by most people is that skid-row bums are our primary problem drinkers, although actually they make up only 3 to 5 percent of the nation's alcoholic population. An estimated 96 million Americans, aged fifteen and up, drink—and 9.6 million of them, one out of every ten, are so addicted to alcohol that they are alcoholics. Alcohol abusers shorten their life-spans by ten to twelve years, and, by their drinking, seriously affect, on the average, the lives of four other persons. The drain on the nation's economy amounts to approximately fifteen billion dollars a year. Ten billion of this sum is attributable to lost working time, two billion goes for health and welfare services for the alcoholics and their families, and three billion is spent on property damage and medical expenses.

Alcohol figures in 85 percent of all liver diseases, 40 percent of all peptic ulcers, 18 percent of stomach, lung, and throat cancers, and many other ailments are related to its abuse, according to Dr. Nelson Bradley, medical director of the alcoholism treatment program at Lutheran General Hospital in Park Ridge, Illinois. This hospital has developed a twenty-eight-day in-hospital treatment program with a ten-week follow-up of patients that boasts 70 to 80 percent success in arresting alcoholism.

Alcohol is a depressant that acts on the central nervous system, primarily the brain. Instead of being digested, it is absorbed directly into the bloodstream where it travels to the brain, and behaves there much like the proverbial bull in the china shop. It interferes with brain chemistry and partially or completely turns off memory, judgment, learning ability, reaction time, coordination, and, if drinking is prolonged, consciousness. Should a drinker consume thirty to thirty-five ounces of alcohol in a relatively short time, the brain centers that control heartbeat and breathing are so depressed that the drinker may die.

Even light or moderate drinkers may be exposing themselves to irreversible damage with each drink they take. Cirrhosis of the liver was, until recently, thought to be the most serious disease of the heavy drinker. New research shows that alcohol damages or destroys cells in the brain, muscles, heart, and other organs. It is now believed that each drink destroys some brain cells—and brain cells, once destroyed, can never be replaced.

Even the abstainers, those who do not drink at all, are not immune to the wide swath alcohol cuts through the fabric of American life. Some experts estimate that one out of every ten cars you meet on the highway may be driven by an alcoholic.* Alcohol is blamed for half our annual highway fatalities; for those between the ages of sixteen and twenty-four, the death rate of alcohol-related traffic fatalities rises to 60 percent. Forty

* Statistics about drinking and alcoholism vary considerably depending on the nature and scope of the surveys and studies involved. For example, the *New York Motorist*, official publication of the Automobile Club of New York, stated in a recent article that "one out of every 15 drinking Americans (about three-fourths of our fellow citizens indulge) is an alcoholic."

percent of the annual five million arrests in this country are related to mis-use of alcohol, and one-third of all murder victims have significant amounts of alcohol in their blood at the time of autopsy.

Although alcohol consumption increased by 20 percent during the 1960s, not all who use it do so to the point of abuse. Experts in the field of alcoholism concur that it is a complex disease involving physical, psychological, and social factors. Research has discounted the myths that alcoholism stems from allergic reactions, that it is inherited, or that it is due to an "alcoholic personality." The key to whether or not a person becomes an alcoholic is largely a psychological one, these experts agree, and the alcoholic is the person who is unable or unwilling to tolerate ten-sion or stress. For these people, alcohol is used increasingly to dull the pain and stress of life.

Noise as a Stressor

Silence is of utmost importance in yoga. Only in silence can meditation take place, and meditation is a necessary avenue to samadhi, union with the Infinite. Silence, unfortunately, is a rare commodity in contemporary America.

We're all familiar with the tense, jittery feeling produced by prolonged noise, and noise is now becoming known as one of our primary stressors. In fact, Dr. Eric Frankel, writing in the *British Medical Journal*, feels that many of the young people who take drugs or join violent protest move-ments do so because they are being brainwashed by noise. He states that the noise from pop-music groups, places of work, and traffic have all reached the saturation point. When the stimulus of television, movies, and comics is added to these accumulations, youngsters' brains are stimulated beyond the brain's capacity to absorb it, and the doctor feels that drugs are an attempt to escape.

Even our homes, which should be a haven from the world's clatter, are alarmingly noisy. All family members suffer physically and psychologically because of it. A recent study by the University of Wisconsin Department of Environmental Design claims that noise in the home contributes to breakdowns in family communications, tired-mother syndrome (a worn-out, irritable, and depressed feeling), hyperactivity and short attention span in children—and even divorce.

Most housewives, particularly those with small children, have what I call the "awful hour," a time when meal preparation conflicts with after-school exuberance and after-school snacks, when television or stereo blares away, a time when there seems to be generally too much commotion to tolerate. Many kitchen accidents seem to occur during the "awful hour," and they may be caused by the harassed mother's subconscious attempt to escape from more racket than her nervous system can bear.

Noise has only recently come into its own as a recognized stressor, though loud noises have been known to be harmful to hearing. In the early 1960s pioneer noise researcher Dr. Samuel Rosen, a New York otologist, determined that prolonged exposure to excessive noise not only causes progressive hearing loss but also has a measurable effect on the circulatory system, causing constriction of the arteries, increased rate of heartbeat, and increased flow of adrenaline into the bloodstream.

Another noise researcher conducting experiments in the early sixties was Dr. Gerd Jansen, who was then with the Max Planck Institute in Dortmund, Germany. The subjects of Dr. Jansen's research were 1,005 West German workmen in steel mills and ironworks; 665 of the workmen had the noisiest possible jobs, and 340 worked at quiet jobs.

Dr. Jansen discovered that at 70 decibels, the equivalent of the noise level of traffic on a relatively quiet city street, the autonomic nervous system begins to react. The autonomic nervous system controls such involuntary responses as heartbeat, temperature, digestion, and respiration, and at that 70-decibel level it was noted that a narrowing of the arteries took place. This raises the diastolic blood pressure and lessens the supply of blood to the heart.

Even more dramatic results were produced as the noise levels increased: "dilation of the pupils, drying of the mouth and tongue, loss of skin color, contraction of leg, abdomen and chest muscles, sudden excess production of adrenalin, stoppage of the flow of gastric juices, and excitation of the heart. These effects were automatic, unaffected by the subject's health, his annoyance, or whether he was accustomed to noise on his job," according to the report of this research published in *Reader's Digest*.

Resilient and adaptive as the human body is, it shows no sign of an ability to become conditioned to noise. The human response to noise is affected not only by the loudness, pitch, and duration of the sound but also by the hearer's own physical and mental state. Some people are simply able to tolerate noise better than others; it is still a physical stressor for them, but for those who find it particularly painful it is both a physical and a psychological stressor.

Noise research conducted since the early sixties reinforces and extends the findings of Dr. Rosen and Dr. Jansen. Dr. Chauncey Leake, of the University of California, San Francisco, states that excessive noise adversely affects the nervous, endocrine, and reproductive systems and may damage unborn children. New Zealand's Dr. A. W. Liley, the world's foremost authority on unborn babies, in a 1972 speech in Chicago called attention to the problem of noise in relation to the unborn: "The fetus does not live in a padded, unchanging cocoon, a state of total sensory deprivation, but in a plastic, reactive structure which buffers and filters, perhaps distorts but does not eliminate the outside world. Nor is the fetus himself inert and stuporous, but active and responsive."

Even those who like loud noise, music for instance, are stressed by it. Dr. Leake defines noise as "stressful or unwanted sound." Being unaware of the stress, even enjoying it as loud music, an exuberant football crowd, or the roar of the ocean, does not minimize the damage done by the noise stressor. When the exposure is prolonged, the result is assault and insult to our bodies and nervous systems.

Sound is measured in decibels (db). Zero decibels is the faintest sound that one can hear—the softest breath or the barely audible rustle of a leaf. The decibel scale is a logarithmic scale, and for every ten-degree increase on this scale, the pressure of the sound increases by ten times. In other words, a 20-db sound has ten times more pressure than a 10-db sound.

Most noise experts agree that continual exposure to any sound level over the 50–60-db range, the range of normal conversation, is harmful and that at 120 db the sound is deafening and physically painful. The rating scale below lists the sound range in decibels and qualifies these ranges:

> 100–140 db—deafening
> 80–100 db—very loud
> 60–80 db—loud
> 40–60 db—faint
> 0–20   db—very faint

The decibel rating of the sounds you encounter daily, even in your own home, may surprise you. Listed below are the ratings of some sounds that you probably hear frequently.

Sounds	Decibels
Jet airport	120
Noisy kitchen	100
Power lawn mower	95
Food blender	90
Noisy exhaust fan	90
Vacuum cleaner	87
Garbage-disposal unit	80
Dishwasher	70
Normal conversation	60
Whisper	30
Breathing	10

A University of Wisconsin report on home noise states that it is not unusual to have readings above 100 db during peak activity periods in the average kitchen. They also state that 100 db is too much noise for anyone's physical well-being. Armed with these figures, the housewife would be well advised to plan the use of noisy appliances in such a way that the noise level is spread throughout the day rather than concentrated all at once.

Because our environment is so noisy, we frequently tune out some of it so that we are not consciously aware of it. Few people are aware of furnace noise or the hum of the refrigerator or any number of other sounds that permeate our lives. Even though we are unaware of them, they still provide stress. This has been proved by scientific studies on the effect of low-level noise on sleeping subjects, which show that noises that do not awaken the sleeper still stress him to the point of being tired the next day.

Alternatives

We live in a fast-paced, hectic environment in which environmental stressors such as noise and air pollution are heaped upon the already monumental pile of stressors that confront our citizenry. Yoga is not going to eliminate stress from your life, but the stretching exercises will reduce a great deal of tension that is caused by stress. Yoga won't guarantee that you don't develop one of the stress-related diseases, but it instills a greater appreciation—almost a feeling of reverence—for the human body, mind, and spirit, a feeling that might discourage self-destructive habits of diet and thinking. And without the added burden of self-induced stressors such as alcohol, coffee, and cigarettes, many of our inherited weak spots may not give way and provide easy access for the stress-linked diseases.

With better self-understanding through yoga, you can learn to recognize how many of your attitudes about yourself, and many of your self-destructive habits, have been programmed into you since infancy. Once you recognize the situation, you have taken a giant stride toward correcting it. While you cannot control or change what has happened in your past, only you can control how you react to it now.

And through yoga, you may see life in a different perspective that will change your sense of values, lessening the hold of material possessions and changing your life-style into a more serene existence. You needn't take this possibility at face value, but do remember that much of yoga must be experienced to be believed. Give it, and yourself, a chance.

7

YOGA FOR BEAUTY

Beauty *is* only skin deep, and we all know people whose plainness, or even downright homeliness, is insignificant because of a magnetic personality, wit, kindness, or a host of other endearing qualities. Character attributes are undoubtedly of greater importance than physical beauty, but your physical appearance is still the first impression you present to the world. I think all people owe it to themselves, and to those around them, to look their very best.

Not everyone is endowed with a glamorous Hollywood-type face and figure, but everyone can make the most of his or her natural physical endowments. If a look in the mirror leaves you less than ecstatic, take stock of your assets and liabilities, then employ yoga methods to improve the total picture.

Analyzing Yourself

Stand in front of a full-length mirror, preferably nude, and take a good look at yourself without pulling in the tummy, correcting the posture, or otherwise distorting the way your body is arranged as you stand naturally. Comforting as it is to make these corrective adjustments, you will not get a true picture of your figure assets and liabilities unless you judge your figure as it actually appears when you are in repose. This is also true when analyzing your face. I think everyone has been shocked at the results of a photograph taken when he or she is unaware of it and hasn't presented the best face or angle to the camera.

Use a hand mirror, and check your body from all angles. Take your measurements, date them, and file for future reference. Keep in mind that yoga practice may well decrease your measurements without affecting your weight. Those who approach yoga practice seriously, and devote at least thirty to forty minutes a day to it, should see definite changes in their figure in eight weeks. The following checklist will help you pinpoint problem areas, and the remainder of this chapter offers suggestions for improvement.

FIGURE ANALYSIS

Body Characteristics	Good to Excellent	Needs Improvement
Posture		
Head juts forward		
Slumping shoulders		
Dowager's hump		
Protruding abdomen		
Swayback		
Toes point in or out		
Facial area		
Wrinkles		
Skin tone		
Facial tension		
Expression		
Bustline		
Sagging		
Underdeveloped		
Overdeveloped		
Arms		
Heavy upper arms		
Waistline		
Too large		
Fat at back of waist		
Fat at sides of waist		
Protruding abdomen		
Hips		
Too large		
Out of proportion to rest of body		
Sagging buttocks		
Legs and thighs		
Large thighs		
Saddlebags		
Underdeveloped calves		
Thick ankles		

Set Your Goals

After analyzing the pluses and minuses of your total picture, determine what changes would improve this picture, and incorporate corrective exercises into your daily practice to bring about these changes. For example, if heavy thighs are your main problem, work through the Basic Lesson Plan listed on page 84, but add to it some or all of the exercises specifically designed to trim heavy thighs. Whatever the problem areas, there are corrective or normalizing exercises to help overcome them.

The importance of visualization can't be stressed too strongly when you are trying to produce figure changes. If visualization is difficult for you, it may help to get out a photograph of yourself that you find flattering and recall that photograph mentally several times each day. This is particularly effective if the problem you are trying to eliminate is wrinkling in the facial area. Keep mentally seeing your face without the wrinkles. However, be realistic—if you're in the senior-citizen category, some lines lend character to the face, and a total lack of them would appear unnatural.

If visualization is a new dimension for you, please don't dismiss it as nonsense until you've given it a fair trial. Remember that what you can believe you can achieve.

Posture—Its Importance in Beauty and Aging

Aging is a dirty word in contemporary America, where the median age is twenty-eight. This means that half the people in this country are twenty-eight or under, an unsettling thought for the other half.

Mental attitude and continued activity figure heavily in the fight against age, a theory remarkably demonstrated by such ageless notables as Pablo Casals, ninety-six; Marc Chagall, eighty-six; and Helen Hayes, a lovely lady of seventy-two. And reportedly, Lowell Thomas remains an avid skier, though he is in his eighty-first year.

Today's clothing styles are such that people who stay in shape physically need not be labeled old unless they choose to be. And the cosmetics industry is a willing ally in minimizing the visible effects of the ongoing years. But there is one dead giveaway that Father Time is winning the battle, even if proper weight is maintained, clothing is youthful, and the face unlined. For those who literally shoulder the burden of years, the resulting bad posture gives an aged look.

And we all, consciously or subconsciously, use the posture of others as a yardstick in judging them. Bad posture presents a "loser" image, just as surely as erect carriage labels one a "winner." Posture also has health ramifications. Rounded shoulders cramp the heart and lungs and decrease the amount of vital oxygen carried to all of the cells and the brain. A protruding abdomen disturbs the normal placement of the stomach, kidneys, and the reproductive and elimination systems.

Posture is best analyzed from the side. In perfect posture a vertical line down the side of the body would run from the earlobe, through the shoulder, on through the hipbone, and terminate at the anklebone. You will need someone to help you check this side view; if no one is available, try the old standard posture test of backing up against a wall, place your heels against the wall, and you should also touch the wall at the buttocks, shoulders, and back of the head. If you can get your fist between your body and the wall at the small of your back, it indicates that you are swaybacked. The space at the back of the waist should be about the thickness of your flattened hand.

Exercises for Correcting Swayback and Protruding Abdomen

In the swaybacked individual the pelvis is tilted down and backward instead of up and forward, and the abdomen protrudes. This condition frequently leads to severe lower-back pain. Exercises to correct swayback also reduce the tummy area. To eliminate or minimize swayback, try the following:

1. Pull in the abdomen, which tilts the pelvis forward as it should be. Do this several times during the day.

2. Lie on your back on a smooth-surfaced floor, arms at your sides, palms flat. Bend your knees until you can place the small of your back against the floor, with feet twelve to eighteen inches apart. Now slowly slide the feet away from your body, concentrating on keeping the small of your back pressed against the floor. Do this several times a day, and you will find that the small of your back remains against the floor progressively longer. This is also a good tummy flattener.

3. The Arch posture, both variations, shown on page 145.

4. An additional abdominal exercise is Uddiyana, shown on page 182.

Round Shoulders and Dowager's Hump

1. The Blade, shown on page 132.
2. Shoulder Pulls, shown on page 131.
3. Shoulder Flexing, shown on page 133.
4. The Cobra, shown on page 105, both variations.

5. The Bow, shown on page 110.
6. The Wheel, shown on page 127.
7. The Back Push-up, shown on page 157.
8. The Camel, shown on page 135.
9. The Chest Expansion, shown on page 157.

In addition to poor posture, another cause of dowager's hump is that calcium is withdrawn from the spine after menopause and the body of the vertebrae lose size and may even collapse. To minimize the chance of this occurring, women should be certain to obtain at least the same amount of calcium that is found in a quart of milk each day. This can be whole milk, skim milk, or nonfat dry milk products, which are often used in cooking. Calcium tablets may also be taken, as is commonly done in pregnancy, to prevent a calcium deficiency.

In addition to the foregoing exercises, any that strengthen the back and abdominal muscles are safeguards against this unsightly deformity.

The Face

The aging process has been called a series of small collapses. The hardest to bear, for most women at least, is the loss of a young-looking face. Dry, wrinkled skin is a dead giveaway that youth, if not fleeing, is at least tugging at the leash.

Much criticism has been leveled at the cosmetics industry to the effect that advertising claims are exaggerations. The current ecology boom is producing many new cosmetics firms that use natural products such as cucumbers and strawberries and various vitamin combinations. One of the popular ecological cosmetic items is a combination of natural oils that is used to keep the skin moist and relatively unwrinkled. Do-it-yourself types can make this at home from ingredients found in health-food stores at much less cost and feel creative at the same time.

One problem with regular cosmetic oils and creams is that the ingredients are not listed and many people suffer allergic reactions to them. The following formula should be allowed to remain on the face and neck for at least ten minutes and should then be removed with the astringent. The astringent ingredients are inexpensive drugstore items.

CLEOPATRA'S FORMULA

3 tablespoons safflower oil
3 tablespoons seasame oil
2 tablespoons sunflower oil
2 tablespoons avocado oil

2 tablespoons peanut oil
1 tablespoon olive oil
1 tablespoon wheat-germ oil
5 drops of perfume or oil of rose geranium

ASTRINGENT

¾ cup rose water	Pinch of alum powder
¼ cup witch hazel	¼ teaspoon glycerin
1 teaspoon honey	½ teaspoon spirit of camphor
½ teaspoon white vinegar	½ teaspoon extract of mint

Two primary reasons for aging of the facial skin are lack of circulation to this area and the pull of gravity, which constantly tugs at the facial tissues. Those yoga students who do the Headstand, the Half Shoulder Stand, and the Pose of Tranquillity will discover that they increase facial circulation and reverse the pull of gravity. The Lion (see photo of this posture on page 180) also increases facial circulation.

Yoga has been said to "freeze one's age," but no one with or without yoga can expect to live to extreme old age with a completely unlined face. However, wrinkles and lines are not the same thing. Wrinkles are an actual crumpling of the skin, usually from neglect, faulty diet, sudden weight loss, and tension. Lines, on the other hand, reflect character, personality, and experience in life. Change is inevitable in the human face, because every time we smile, frown, or yawn, the skin is creased, thus creating lines. These movements are repeated thousands of times in a lifetime, and as the face loses its baby fat, these lines deepen. If the skin is kept fresh and healthy and the muscle tone remains firm, these lines of maturity add strength and character to the face.

For those who have not yet mastered the Headstand, the following exercises will increase circulation in the all-important facial area, helping to prevent wrinkles.

1. Stand with feet slightly apart, inhale, and fall forward from the waist as you exhale. The upper body, head, and arms should be as limp as a rag doll. Just let yourself flop. Hold for a count of ten, and return to standing position; repeat five times.

2. Again standing with feet slightly apart, inhale, and flop to the right side as you exhale; repeat in center position, then on the left side. Perform this cycle several times.

3. Stand with feet apart, and place palms on the backs of your thighs. Inhale, and while exhaling, run the hands down the backs of the legs, trying to grasp the ankles. Try to pull the head between the knees, keeping the legs straight.

4. Stand with legs apart, hands clasped on top of the head with fingers interlaced, palms up. Inhale, and stretch the palms toward the ceiling. Exhale as you bend from the thigh joints until clasped palms rest on the floor. The knees must be kept straight, but the farther apart the feet, the easier it is to reach the floor.

While performing these exercises, visualize your face as you wish it to be. If some wrinkling has already occurred, mentally picture your face without wrinkles. Don't let your thoughts wander. Keep your ideal facial image firmly in mind.

Facial Tension

One of the results of facial tension and general inner tension is chronic unconscious frowning, and the evidence of this is a vertical line—or lines—that form between the eyebrows. This is a hard habit to overcome because people are unaware they are doing it. While we are trying to develop inner resources in yoga, sometimes an assist is needed, and this is one such case.

There is a commercial product called Frownies, available in drugstores, which consists of a triangular paste-on piece of paper that helps eliminate these frown lines. Used during sleep, they smooth out these lines; during the day they make the person aware of how often he or she frowns. If they are not available in your area, cut some out of the brown gummed paper used for wrapping packages for mailing, or write to the manufacturer, The B and P Company, P.O. Box 2632, Cleveland, Ohio. The cost is two dollars for four hundred Frownies.

Wrinkles and Smoking

You may very well have come a long way, baby, as one cigarette commercial suggests, but the journey has not been entirely to your advantage. Approximately 30.5 percent of the nation's adult women smoke, and smoking and premature facial wrinkling go hand in hand. A California survey conducted by a medical doctor on more than one thousand subjects found that premature wrinkling is related to duration and intensity of smoking in both men and women. In the forty-to-forty-nine age group smokers were found to be as wrinkled as nonsmokers who were twenty years older.

Probably the biggest complaint most people express when contemplating the abandonment of cigarettes is the fear of weight gain. Most doctors maintain that this is the result of new nonsmokers filling the void by eating more food. Now, however, Dr. Neil Solomon, Secretary of Health and Mental Hygiene for the State of Maryland and an assistant professor of psychiatry and behavioral sciences at the Johns Hopkins University School of Medicine in Baltimore, and many of his colleagues in the profession confirm that stopping smoking *does* contribute to added weight, though not merely because of the propensity to eat more.

According to Dr. Solomon, the nicotine in cigarettes stimulates the metabolism, and when a person stops smoking, his metabolism decreases its efficiency by 10 percent while the body is adjusting to the lack of nicotine. This adjustment period takes approximately three months.

After the three-month adjustment period the body has become accustomed to the lack of nicotine, and the metabolism returns to normal. Unless the virtuous nonsmoker *cuts* his food intake during this period, he can expect to gain 10 percent of his total weight while this adjustment is taking place. As a preventive measure, food intake must be cut by 10 percent, or the amount of exercise normally performed must be increased accordingly.

For those who wish to eliminate this expensive and unhealthy habit, yoga offers a few helpful hints. The first of these is autosuggestion, which is a form of programming your subconscious. To do this, mentally repeat to yourself, "I am a nonsmoker." Practice doing this several times a day, particularly as you are drifting off to sleep at night. If you intend to quit on some specific date in the future, such as the first day of the next month or the beginning of the new year, begin now to change your self-image to that of a nonsmoker, and don't be concerned about the fact that you continue to smoke. Eventually the resolution will take root in your subconscious and be actualized in your behavior.

This technique may sound a bit naïve to some people, but it worked for S. I. Hayakawa, the famous California educator. In three months, using this technique alone, he kicked a pack-and-a-half-a-day habit of some thirty years standing.

Many people trying to quit complain that they become nervous when they refrain from smoking. Yoga has an answer for that, too—deep, rhythmic breathing. To do this, as already explained in Chapter 3, extend the abdomen as you inhale to a count of four, hold your breath for two counts, exhale while pulling the abdomen in for a count of four, and hold the lungs empty for two counts. Continue this routine until you feel calm and in control again. This form of breathing increases the oxygen in the system and calms the nerves. If you happen to suffer from insomnia, it helps combat that complaint as well.

Facial Expression Is Key to Personality

The eyes have been called the windows of the soul, but the mouth is far more revealing of one's personality and attitudes. Frowning uses twice as many muscles as smiling and creates facial tension. A smile relaxes the face and eases tension. Photographers used to ask their subjects to say "cheese" to achieve a pleasant facial expression. The word "serene" does the same thing, and its effect is more than physical. Say the word quietly to yourself a few times, and notice the calming effect it has on your mental and spiritual outlook.

The Waistline

A bulging waistline is one of the most unattractive and aging of figure faults. Besides being unattractive, fat around the waist is one of the standard indicators of obesity.

Take the pinch test, and see how you measure up, literally. With thumb and index finger grasp the skin around the waist. If the thickness of this pinched skin measures more than one-half inch, it is an indication of excess weight. Though this test may seem severe, keep in mind that obesity is present when a person is 10 to 15 percent over his or her ideal weight in the standard weight tables prepared by life-insurance companies.

To trim the waistline, try the following exercises:
1. The Side Slip, shown on page 170.
2. The Triangle, both variations, shown on pages 129–130.
3. The Lying Twist, both variations, shown on page 164.

For fat at the back of the waistline, one of the hardest places to reduce, try:
1. The Wheel, shown on page 127.
2. The Bow, shown on page 110.
3. The Camel, shown on page 135.
4. The Cat Stretch, shown on page 158.

The Bustline

No part of the human female anatomy has received so much attention as the bustline, one of the yardsticks of female pulchritude. Strangely, the breast is largely fatty tissue. Seemingly geared to heredity, fat on some people accumulates in this area creating an ample bust, while on others it accumulates in other areas and is considered a problem at that point. Everything is relative.

For women with small busts, improved muscle tone of the pectoral muscles that hold the breasts up or allow them to sag will bolster the general appearance of the bustline. Many yoga asanas contribute to this, the best being Variation #2 of the Cobra, shown on page 107. The Headstand is also noted for improving body symmetry, frequently reducing the hips and seemingly increasing the size of the bustline.

For the woman whose bust is larger than desired, a general weight loss is advisable if she is overweight. Unfortunately, neither yoga nor medical science has come up with much help beyond this. If this is your physical hang-up, be consoled that many women would gladly trade places with you.

Heavy Upper Arms

Increasing years, inactivity, and extra pounds often conspire to produce unattractively heavy upper arms. This is frequently accompanied by a lessening of strength in the arms generally. The following exercises will alleviate both conditions:
1. The Cobra, Variation #2, shown on page 107.
2. The Swan, shown on page 175.
3. Shoulder Pulls, shown on page 131.

Hips

The area between the knees and the waistline is a problem for many women, and many hip exercises also aid thighs and upper legs, and some exercises meant specifically for the thighs also improve the hipline in the process. You will be able to judge which parts of your body are being affected by the recommended exercises after you have done them a few times. The best exercises for hips and sagging buttocks are:
1. The Half Lotus, shown on page 166.
2. The Cat Stretch, shown on page 158.

Legs and Thighs

Most women have at least one figure problem, and for many it is heavy thighs. Unfortunately, the female body structure predisposes many to heaviness through the hip and thigh areas. Fat accumulates most readily in areas that are moved infrequently, as in the saddlebag section of the upper outer thigh. Even teen-agers, many of whom are willow slim, are plagued with disproportionately thick thighs.

In decades past, some of this heaviness was camouflaged by constricting girdles and long hemlines. Today's accent on naturalness goes hand in hand with the yoga concept of conditioning one's body so that girdles and other illusion-inducing apparel are unnecessary.

Many women escape the problem of heavy thighs through their teens and twenties only to find it a most unwelcome condition in their thirties. Women whose jobs or life-styles are somewhat sedentary are particularly prone to this sort of "spreading." Even the housewife with small children who spends hours each day in housework and strenuous child-oriented activities finds that the kind of exercise she gets, though fatiguing, doesn't do much for her figure.

The following leg and thigh exercises can reshape these areas almost magically. Most yoga postures benefit more than one area, so you will find improvements elsewhere also.

1. The Camel (Pelvic Stretch), shown on page 135.
2. The Sitting Five-Step, shown on page 120.
3. The Side Leg Raises, shown on pages 153–154.
4. The Deep Lunge, shown on page 160.
5. The Side Slip, shown on page 170.
6. The Triangle, shown on page 129.

Feet and Ankles

Everyone knows each detail of his or her own face, but this interest diminishes greatly when it comes to the feet. Unless they've given you trouble, when was the last time you really thought about your feet?

The foot is a marvelously engineered part of the body, consisting of twenty-six bones and a network of muscles, ligaments, nerves, and blood vessels. Besides providing a most efficient method of getting from one place to another, feet also are essential to the balance of the body and act as shock absorbers so that walking and running do not jolt the all-important spinal column.

Shoes, which restrict normal foot movement, and the aging process tend to reduce circulation in the foot. One obvious result of lack of circulation is swelling of the feet and ankles. People of any age will be amazed at the increased circulation provided by the series of foot exercises shown on page 000. The effect is surprisingly pleasant for everyone and is especially beneficial to the elderly.

Lopsidedness

Have you ever stopped to think that life tends to make us all unbalanced, or at least a bit lopsided? From childhood on we have been forced to become right- or left-handed because of school desks, scissors, and baseball bats, among other things. This imbalance is carried into adult life by refrigerator doors designed for right or left hand, golf clubs, and all the other things that are customarily done with either the right or left hand. In view of this situation it is not surprising that people's bodies develop disproportionately, one side being larger or stronger than the other. You will notice when performing asanas that it is always easier to move one side of the body than the other. This is particularly true of the muscles in the arms and back. Rishi's Twist, shown on page 151, counteracts this imbalance by providing an intense stretch for arms and back muscles.

Avoiding Cycles

The average person goes through several distinct physical cycles during a year. Typically, the first of each year finds most people burdened with extra holiday poundage, due to little exercise and a diet inadequate in fresh fruits and vegetables. The added weight remains, camouflaged under layers of winter clothing, until those first warm days of early spring hint that the excesses can't be hidden indefinitely.

Next comes a frantic attempt to jog, diet, exercise, or somehow manipulate the body into acceptable shape for summer's more revealing clothing and way of life. Many of these crash attempts produce the desired results, but as the years go by, it becomes more and more difficult to break the grip of those bad habits that produced the problem in the first place.

Fall curtails many forms of physical activity, and the vicious circle begins to repeat itself. As the holiday season becomes just another memory, we're again out of shape.

Why not resolve now to plan a physical regime that is constant and moderate instead of being a victim of a sporadic, feast-or-famine way of life? A program of diet and exercise initiated now will keep you in great shape throughout the year. A program of good, healthful living, just like yoga, must be a way of life and not just a sometime thing.

8

REINCARNATION, THE OCCULT, AND ASTROLOGY

Emerson in "Compensation" wrote: "The world looks like a mathematical equation, which, turn it how you will, balances itself. Every secret is told, every crime punished, every wrong redressed, in silence and certainty." He might well have been referring to reincarnation, a basic tenet of yoga.

Emerson believed in reincarnation, as did Walt Whitman, Goethe, Ben Franklin, Mark Twain, Plato, Schopenhauer, Bronson and Louisa May Alcott, Arthur Conan Doyle, and many others. Many of those who disbelieve confuse reincarnation with transmigration of souls, the concept that man returns to earth, after death, in animal form.

Transmigration of souls is a superstition endorsed by many uneducated sects in the East and is a misconception of the true reincarnation principle. Millions of educated people throughout the world believe in reincarnation and guide their lives by means of its ethical principles.

Reincarnation Defined

Reincarnation is the theory that each person's soul is a continuing entity throughout eternity. The soul was not created at birth, nor is it extinguished at the point we know as death. Reincarnation is the evolution of man's soul through many successive lifetimes on earth—sometimes as a man, at other times as a woman, in one life a rich man, and in another a pauper, this time as a black, and the next a member of another race.

This succession of lives is a learning experience for the soul and continues until the soul has reached a state of perfection and can be reunited with God, or the Ultimate Reality.

Part of the reincarnation theory is the law of karma, the law of cause and effect, of action and reaction, or "as ye sow, so shall ye reap." A person's karma is the sum total of all the good and evil he has done in previous lifetimes. Our present condition is the result of what we have made ourselves from our past. Karma is the balance sheet of the soul.

Karma is built up by our every thought, word, and action and by the motivations behind those activities. For example, a person who helps a friend in need would presumably be fashioning good karma. If the service is performed to secure eternal gratitude or personal recognition, however, this negates the good of the action. Motive is all-important. Each person, by his thoughts, words, and actions, becomes the molder of his destiny. Like a boomerang, whatever he wisely or unwisely sets in motion will return to him in full measure.

The concept of reincarnation and karma infers that the moral and spiritual worlds are subject to laws of cause and effect as precise as those governing the physical world. Human suffering is no mere happenstance, but the result of errors in conduct or thinking. The physical and mental inequalities that we glimpse all around us arise from merits and demerits of past life behavior. All pain and limitations are learning experiences for the soul.

Christianity's explanation of human suffering is that man has a soul and that it is immortal. Suffering is a test given us by God, and depending on how that challenge is met, we are rewarded by heaven or hell. Reincarnation is somewhat the same concept, except it spreads the punishment or reward over several lifetimes instead of just one.

Paramahansa Yogananda, in *Autobiography of a Yogi*, had this to say on the subject:

> Many Biblical passages reveal that the law of reincarnation was understood and believed. In fact, the early Christian church accepted the doctrine of reincarnation, which was expounded by the Gnostics and by numerous church fathers, including the celebrated Origen and St. Jerome. The doctrine was first declared a heresy in 553 A.D. by the Second Council of Constantinople. At that time, too many Christians thought the doctrine of reincarnation afforded man too ample a stage of time and space to encourage him to strive for immediate salvation.

The Occult Boom

We are currently seeing a revival of interest in spiritual matters and in the occult, not only in the United States but throughout the world. Nearly every newspaper carries an astrological horoscope column, Ouija board sales have skyrocketed, and on the 1971 *Apollo 14* moon flight, Astronaut Edgar Mitchell conducted experiments in mental communication with four earthbound persons. Occult books and bookstores abound, and crystal balls are as commonplace in the suburbs as in the séance. The occult, of course, has always had its devotees. The word means "hidden" and denotes hidden knowledge or unexplainable phenomena. What is unique about the occult takeoff of the 1970s compared to earlier periods of popularity is the type of person involved. Previous participants were generally bored or eccentric old ladies who attended fake séances in an effort to keep tabs on a departed spouse. Current psychic searchers, however, include some scientists, doctors, lawyers, educators, and theologians, along with the omnipresent lunatic fringe, which probably accounts for the fact that the occult has never been considered quite respectable. Proponents of the occult who contribute much to its lunacy image are, generally speaking, individuals who have made a poor adjustment to the here and now and turn to this less tangible form of reality as a cop-out or because they are misfits in day-to-day life.

Occult Categories

The occult binge of the seventies can be loosely divided into four primary categories—satanism, witchcraft, prophecy, and spiritualism—and there are benign as well as malignant factions in these groups. In its most innocuous form the satanists are pure pleasure-seekers, striving for material possessions and personal sensual pleasures. They don't actually hurt anyone, but if the purpose of life is spiritual progression, their lives will manifest little in the way of spiritual growth. Their more perverted factions are involved in such sordid activities that they contribute to some of our shocking headlines.

Witchcraft also divides into two groups—black and white—and the only distinction between the two is motivation. The white witches, of whom Sybil Leek is our best-known advocate, use their ancient rituals and power for good, such as healing and harmony. Black witchcraft, on the other hand, is concerned with devil dolls, hexes, and other harmful ritualistic ceremonies.

Prophecy is the basis behind the astrology boom and also accounts for the renewed interest in tarot cards, Ouija, and the I Ching. Our universal interest in what the future holds assures rapt audiences and readers for such psychics as Jeane Dixon and Kreskin who profess the ability to see what lies ahead. Nostradamus, the sixteenth-century physician and astrologer, still has a following, and Edgar Cayce, the seer of Virginia Beach, who died in 1945, hypoed our latent interest in this field to its current high degree of attention. Even the conservative, stable element of our population is turned on when a hunch proves accurate, and recent research proving that successful businessmen have higher measurable amounts of ESP seems to be giving the nod of approval to the expanded use of our senses.

The fourth segment of the occult field is spiritualism, which is the most closely linked to the concept of reincarnation. Assuming that the spirit does survive bodily death, spiritualists work through mediums to contact the spirits of those who have passed over. Spiritualists also work in the field of healing and counseling, and they believe that we all have "spirit guides" who are always present to guide and advise us, this advice coming through to our consciousness as intuition.

Some manifestations of the accuracy of prophecy and spiritualism seem to defy the laws of chance or mere coincidence and are being seriously probed by scientists. It may be that the scientific approach may someday shed light on these occult subjects, bringing our body of natural laws sufficiently up-to-date to explain these phenomena. Even without the substantiation of science, the occult will always fascinate a good many people.

Published interviews with noted historian, philosopher, and author Arnold Toynbee on the structure of our life may explain part of the fascination we have with the occult subjects. Mr. Toynbee believes we are now in the midst of World War III, not a war between nations, but a different kind of war, which has on one side human technology and on the other, human personality. He sees this war as man's struggle to save his personality from destruction by our tremendous technological society—people in revolt against being treated as impersonal numbers, punched onto a card, instead of as human beings.

The progressive depersonalization to which he alludes may well explain the appeal of an astrological horoscope. No two horoscopes are exactly alike, and it can be a comforting thought that although you're a statistic at work, the sun, moon, and all the planets see you as a distinct and separate entity, and their combined forces interact in your life in a completely unique fashion. There's no one in the world quite like you from an astrological standpoint. Spiritualism, with those friendly personal spirit guides, thus can seem appealing in an increasingly impersonal world.

On the surface there seems to be nothing wrong with a healthy interest in the occult. And there really isn't any harm, as long as this interest *is* healthy. Problems arise when individuals become so immersed in the occult world, or the spirit world, that they lose contact with the world of people, with what is going on in contemporary society. Balance is important in yoga, and in all of life, in fact, but it's absolutely vital when dealing with esoteric subjects.

Varying Concepts of Reincarnation

Like most people seriously involved in yoga, I do believe in reincarnation. I believe that the way I look, my personality, abilities, interests, and basic character are the result of many previous lives. But I also believe that the life I am leading now is my most important concern. There are a few people who claim to remember past lives, but the vast majority of us do not, and I strongly feel that we do not remember because we are not spiritually mature enough to be able to handle this knowledge.

Recently I heard an account of a woman who was regressed under hypnosis, in an attempt to learn about past lives. This regression was performed before a group of friends, and during the course of the hypnotic session it was learned that the woman had been married to a particular man in the group during a lifetime around the time of the Civil War. Unbelievable as it may seem, this woman then divorced the husband she had chosen in this lifetime to marry her supposed former husband. This is an example of how belief in a spiritually uplifting doctrine can be misinterpreted, and in the process, becomes extremely disruptive to personal stability.

Reincarnation teaches that in the afterlife we are not "up there" or "down there," but right here in the same general location as our known physical world. Those who have passed over can see us, but we cannot see them, because they possess bodily vehicles that are of a different frequency of vibration than ours. Comfortingly, those who die old or infirm seem to have the ability to mentally restructure their bodies back to a period when that body was comfortable. Everything in the afterlife plane is accomplished by thought. Should a spirit wish to see what his family is doing, he can transport himself to where they are located merely by means of the power of thought.

One of the more interesting books on the subject of reincarnation is *A World Beyond*, by Ruth Montgomery. The most unusual facet of this volume is that it was supposedly dictated via automatic writing by Arthur Ford, one of America's most famous mediums, after his death in January, 1971.

The book tells quite specifically what happens at the time of death and after death. We are told that Ford's purpose in dictating this book after death was to substantiate the theory that life does continue after death, and he makes that life sound much more interesting than an afterlife spent winging about, harp in hand. He describes it as a time spent in advanced study and self-evaluation and negates the concept of a judgment day, stressing that we all must judge ourselves when the time comes. Fortunately, we see our lives and our soul qualities from a different perspective on the other side. When we elect to try earth life again, the soul has certain spiritual growth objectives in mind.

The yogalike aspect of this book is its emphasis on the importance of discipline. Ford states that the urge to smoke, drink, or overindulge in sex or food should be overcome during earth life because there are no vehicles in the afterlife to teach discipline.

The woman who changed husbands after regression could have profited by a more serious study of the basics of reincarnation. By her action, she was regressing and losing track of what her soul intended to accomplish during this lifetime. In essence she was repeating a prior experience and one that was probably not in her plans when she took incarnation this time. Getting hung up on prior lives is just what it appears to be—going backward.

The conventional approach to the afterlife proposed by much of Christianity is a pleasant, do-nothing existence in which souls drift around on clouds strumming their harps. My personal inclination, even as a child, has been toward progress, growth, and learning, and the thought of such a dull spiritual climate has never been adequate motivation or reward for trying to be the best person I could be.

Reincarnation's belief, on the other hand, that the afterlife provides opportunity for higher learning, self-study, and integration and assimilation of what is learned is a very exciting prospect. In this concept of afterlife one would have the opportunity to commune with all the souls who share your interests, to pursue those subjects that most fascinate you, and to travel to all parts of the world without the encumbrances of baggage, passport, and finances—and to accomplish this simply by thinking it into existence.

Imagine a rap session with Shakespeare, Michelangelo, Mozart, George Washington, John Kennedy, Clark Gable, Freud, or the great thinkers in any area that grabs your interest! In that life no one directs your interest or study, and you're free to grow and study as much as you wish. It's much like smorgasbording through college taking those subjects that really mean something to you without the necessity of required courses, some of which can be terribly dull.

One of the disadvantages of spiritualism and the efforts of its aficionados to contact the spirits who have passed over is that these contacts distract the work and study that is the purpose of an afterlife. As long as those still in earthly form hang on to their grief, and continually try to maintain contact with their deceased loved ones, they are actually impeding their loved ones' progress in the spirit world.

A good example of this situation is a nationally prominent family whose beautiful, talented daughter was brutally murdered, a crime that remains unsolved. The mother has spent years going from one medium to another trying to contact the daughter and gain information to solve the murder. The mediums she has consulted range from little-known psychics through the most famous of spirit contactors, and the information she has received is of such a personal nature that she is convinced she has been in contact with her daughter. When she presses for the identity of the killer, however, the daughter always replies that she, the daughter, has forgiven him and that the mother should discontinue her search. Regardless of how elevated this mother's motives are, she is still slowing down her daughter's progress on the other side by her persistent efforts and constant need for contact.

All of the contacts with so-called spirits indicate that those spirits prefer their present existence and have no desire to return to the more limited life we enjoy on earth.

Even accounts of people who have expired on the operating table and have been brought back through the marvels of modern medicine indicate that they resented being rescued and after their experience no longer have any fear of death. These spirits or souls of the departed maintain their affectionate ties with earthly family and friends and stay close to them during their period of bereavement, but they're most eager for the mourning to abate so that they can get on with their business on that plane.

Another disadvantage of contacting spirits is that not all of them are good. Having departed mortal life does not automatically convey goodness of character or morals. Those souls that were concerned only with physical gratification on earth are frustrated in the spirit world where they have no opportunity to gratify purely physical desires. These perverted souls occupy very low rungs on the ladder of spiritual evolution, and they welcome earth contacts in order that they may live more or less vicariously through their earth contacts. The recent book *The Exorcist* is a good example of this very dangerous situation.

The Positive Approach to Reincarnation

Reincarnation teaches that when a child is born, it isn't actually starting out anew, but taking up where it left off in previous lives. Even the people in your family and associations are believed to be old acquaintances from previous incarnations. Whatever the tenor of your relationship with them, this time is said to be an intensification of past-life encounters. And if this relationship is not a good one, and the problems aren't resolved, you will probably lock horns with them in future lives.

Viewing interpersonal differences from this vantage point provides a very good reason for utilizing our most mature judgment in relationships with others. With divorce so commonplace and so easy—and humans frequently take the path of least resistance—it might seem much easier to opt for divorce rather than attempt to work out amicable solutions to problems. When you realize, however, that unsolved difficulties will be met later, and they will then be more intense, it may be prudent to settle them now rather than face them later. Putting it off till later lives is like borrowing money at an exorbitantly high interest rate.

The law of reincarnation and karma covers all relationships. Therefore, whatever you mete out to others will be returned to you in full measure in future lives. The child-abusing parent can look forward to being the object of parental brutality, the dishonest may in future lives be deceived, and anyone inflicting torture on humans or animals might well spend an existence without sight or a limb, and so on.

Reincarnation and karma are far from universally accepted theories now, but beliefs do change. Only 419 years ago, Spanish physician Michael Servetus was burned at the stake because his theory of pulmonary circulation, later proved accurate, was contrary to current beliefs. Those who do believe in the law of karma find it good motivation for living the best life possible.

Yoga theory teaches that those who are strongly drawn toward yoga science were probably involved in yoga or related subjects in previous lifetimes, and that there is a "recognition" factor. The Hindu belief in reincarnation is one reason why many natives of India shun the practice of yoga. Although they are familiar with the yoga beliefs and teachings and recognize their merit, there is no compulsion to accept the discipline of yoga "now or never." Since they firmly believe in future lives, "putting off" yoga produces no inner conflict. They simply decide to strive for perfection in another lifetime.

Many who believe in reincarnation feel it works hand in hand with astrology—that people are born at a time when the pull of various planets and the skills, motivation, and emphasis displayed in their charts are most likely to achieve whatever goal was set by the soul for this lifetime.

The Astrology Thing

The occult explosion, and particularly astrology, with its ten million ardent followers and forty million dabblers, is on the way to becoming a contemporary cult that many churches view as a competitor to conventional religion. Viewing this cult as a major American religion, the *Lutheran Witness,* a publication of the Lutheran Church of the Missouri Synod, has researched the subject and concludes that the estimated 1,750 daily horoscope columns in newspapers and the 10,000 full-time and 175,000 part-time astrologers combine to provide more coverage on astrology than that afforded to the churches.

Astrology is also big business. Just the computerized horoscope segment is now more than a 200-million-dollar venture, and then there are the zodiac posters, artwork, jewelry, and toiletries, not to mention the numerous books on the subject in both hard cover and paperback, and the zodiac shops that have sprung up in most major cities.

Furthermore, big business is beginning to use astrology in carrying out its myriad functions. A multimillion-dollar insurance company, National Life Insurance of Vermont, has hired an astrologer to analyze the horoscopes of its employees in order to improve their efficiency. The astrologer will also screen job applicants to predict their suitability. This company turned to astrology because the usual methods of testing personnel proved so unreliable, and company executives hope that astrology will provide them with a better nucleus of staff people.

National Life, which has more than fifteen hundred employees and full-time agents across the nation, has retained astrologer Clifford E. McMillen, an instructor in astrology and ESP for the Dade County (Florida) school system and lecturer at the Miami Museum of Science. Commenting on this assignment in the *National Enquirer*, McMillen said:

> The company is most anxious for me to astrologically chart each prospective salesman over the 2-year period ahead and see if his sales will be hurt by problems of marriage, career or money. I am also analyzing existing salesmen to see, by their astrological charts, who they get along with best—whether, for example, they should be selling to professional people only or to the general public.
>
> The company is also asking me to look at their executives' charts, and those of the legal people they retain. From a person's birth signs, and the position of the planets at the moment he was born, I can tell his ambitions, strong points, weaknesses, motivation, suitability for certain work, stability and other factors.

According to a company spokesman:

> McMillen is surprising us with his results. His analysis of character is amazingly accurate. After five years, 90 percent of insurance salesmen who started with us prove to be failures. This high rate of failure is very costly to us, representing a waste of time, money and effort.

Astrology could be the answer to cutting down on that waste, judging from what I've already seen of McMillen's evaluations. I'm glad we retained him.

McMillen believes the day will come when astrologers will routinely be employed by big companies and states that "two international airlines, Braniff and Swissair, use astrology to tell whether a pilot is going to have a good day or a bad one. Pilots headed for bad days are not allowed to fly," he said.

Meanwhile, psychiatric researchers in Miami have released the results of a two-year study indicating that outbreaks of murder may be triggered by the moon tugging on "biological tides" inside the human body. According to Dr. Arnold L. Lieber, a senior resident in psychiatry at the University of Miami's medical school, the study results show a "scientifically sound relationship" between phases of the moon and the murder rate in Dade County. Lieber also said that a chart of Miami-area homicides over the last fifteen years plotted according to moon phases looks remarkably like a chart of ocean tides.

Using computer programs, Lieber and Dr. Carolyn R. Sherin, of the University of Miami, analyzed nearly nineteen hundred murders that occurred between 1956 and 1970. The data revealed that the county's murder rate began to rise about twenty-four hours before the full moon, reached a peak at full moon, then dropped back before climbing again to a secondary peak at the new moon.

Though the effect of the moon's gravitational pull on humans is small, Lieber stated that it may be enough to touch off emotional instability in "borderline" cases. This instability is reflected in the murder rate, which he terms a reliable measure of the moon's effect on the general population.

Lieber said the makeup of the body itself helped him turn to the concept of "biological tides" to explain the phenomenon. The body is "a microcosm comprising essentially the same elements and in similar proportions as the earth's surface—approximately 80 percent water and 20 percent minerals," he said.

"I feel that eventually we are going to show that any organism, human or animal, is an integral part of the universe and responds to changes like variations in the solar cycle and the lunar cycle."

He added that when the moon and sun are in proper position to exert their greatest gravitational force on the earth, there seems to be an even more marked increase in "ruthless and bizarre" violent crime. During this "maximum tidal force," which occurs about once every fourteen months, Dade County's murder rate rose to four and five murders a day.

Astrology for Nonbelievers

Nearly everyone reads his sun sign horoscope in the newspaper columns, and many find these readings far afield from their actual lives. This is understandable because the newspaper charts must, because of space limitations, assume that everyone was born at 6:00 A.M. Furthermore, they are based only on the sun and do not consider the moon or the other eight planets. To have any real validity, a horoscope chart must be set up for the exact minute and precise location of birth and must take into consideration the placement and relationship between the sun, moon, and planets.

There are many philosophies, religions, and theories containing elements that I feel have value, although I cannot accept the entire body of that belief. If you are one of those who could never take astrology seriously, you can still use it to your advantage as a way of looking at and evaluating how your life is going, in determining the areas that are satisfactory and those that need improvement.

A horoscope chart is erected for the exact minute and location in which a person is born, and once set up can be delineated, or interpreted, in order to understand both character and destiny. Character is determined by the sign (Aries, Taurus, Gemini, Cancer, Leo, Virgo, Libra, Scorpio, Saggitarius, Capricorn, Aquarius, and Pisces) in which planets are located; destiny is determined by the houses in which the planets are located.

Astrology is a complex subject, but an intriguing one. For those who would like to learn more about it, but hesitate to invest in many expensive books that are needed, I would recommend two paperback books to start: *Write Your Own Horoscope*, by Joseph F. Goodavage, and *My World of Astrology*, by Sydney Omarr. If you find that your interest is sustained after reading these, you will then have enough basic knowledge to select the books you need.

9

MIRACLES, MASTERS, AND MEDITATION

My first exposure to yoga came in the 1950s when I read *Autobiography of a Yogi,* by Paramahansa Yogananda, who entered maha samadhi, a yogi's final conscious exit from the body, in Los Angeles, California, on March 7, 1952. The frontispiece of the book included a notarized letter from the mortuary director of Forest Lawn Memorial Park, which is extracted as follows:

> The absence of any visual signs of decay in the dead body of Paramahansa Yogananda offers the most extraordinary case in our experience. . . . No physical disintegration was visible in his body even twenty days after death. . . . No indication of mold was visible on his skin, and no visible desiccation (drying up) took place in the bodily tissues. This state of perfect preservation of a body is, so far as we know from mortuary annals, an unparalleled one. . . . At the time of receiving Yogananda's body, the mortuary personnel expected to observe, through the glass lid of the casket, the usual progressive signs of bodily decay. Our astonishment increased as day followed day without bringing any visible change in the body under observation. Yogananda's body was apparently in a phenomenal state of immutability. . . .
>
> No odor of decay emanated from his body at any time. . . . The physical appearance of Yogananda on March 27, just before the bronze cover of the casket was put into position, was the same as it

had been on March 7th. He looked on March 27 as fresh and as un-
ravaged by decay as he had looked on the night of his death. On
March 27th there was no reason to say that his body had suffered any
visible physical disintegration at all. For these reasons we state again
that the case of Paramahansa Yogananda is unique in our experience.

This would seem to be a miracle, technically defined as "a wonderful
happening that is contrary to or independent of the known laws of nature."
Miracles were commonplace in biblical times, and saints and martyrs
throughout history have reportedly possessed phenomenal powers, but as
our culture produced greater technological and scientific advances, and
correspondingly greater sophistication, miracles and mysticism became
embarrassing and out of phase.

The example of Yogananda's physical incorruptibility has a counterpart
in the Roman Catholic Church. The body of St. Theresa of Avila (1515–
1582), one of the patron saints of Spain, has lain in a church at Alba,
Spain, for four centuries in a state of incorruptibility, accompanied by a
perfume of flowers. During her lifetime she reorganized the Carmelite
Order of Nuns and found her administrative duties hampered by an
uncontrollable talent for levitation. She tried in vain to prevent her "uplifting" experiences, but wrote: "Little precautions are unavailing when the
Lord will have it otherwise." She also had mystical visions, and although
a woman of great wholesomeness of mind and much practical wisdom, her
enemies said that her gifts were the result of possession by evil spirits.

Another of Christianity's levitating saints was seventeenth-century St.
Joseph of Cupertino, whose monastery brothers banished him from serving
at the common table because he wafted toward the ceiling, crockery in
hand. He was possessed of a divine absentmindedness, which, coupled
with his inability to keep his feet on the ground for any length of time,
made him fundamentally unsuited to earthly duties. He found the sight
of holy statues especially elevating, and there are numerous eyewitness
accounts of two saints, one of flesh and one of stone, in rapt communion
far above the ground.

Autobiography of a Yogi recounts the early life and experiences of its
author and presents probably the most comprehensive treatment of the
mystical aspects of yoga and of the powers of Indian masters. Encounters
with miracle workers and spiritual supermen were a necessary part of the
education of the yogi who was to bring a fuller understanding of yoga to
the Western world.

The witnessing of miracles teaches the devotee about maya, a cosmic
illusion. The world as it seems to be is an illusion; it is unreal. The real
world, the world of spirit and miracles, is possible for all who realize that
each individual is a part of God and not a separate entity. The ego-

principle—the I do, I am, I will—is the root cause of maya and delusion. When the ego is stilled, truth enters. The yogic prayer often used in Western yoga classes is a commentary on maya:

> From the unreal to the real,
> From darkness to light,
> From Death to immortality.
>   Om, Shanti, Shanti, Shanti.*

All miracles are possible for a fully illumined master, although each is unique and has a specific purpose in this life. An accurate description of a master, or saint, is difficult because no two are alike. A master is one who realizes himself as the omnipresent soul, not the body man, nor the ego. Each master reflects God in his own way—surely saints would not be cast from similar molds in a universe so diverse that each set of fingerprints and each snowflake has its own identity. Some masters perform miracles while others shun a display of superphysical powers. There are masters who pass their entire lives in quiet seclusion, and there are others whose purpose in this incarnation is to touch the masses, to teach, and to train disciples.

God-illumined masters are not bound by our conventional concept of time and space, and the past, present, and future are easily accessible to them. Saints discern the minutiae of one's life with the same facile ease that they exhibit in recalling, or foretelling, our triumphs and tragedies. These abilities assault the known laws of our universe, the laws that have been discovered by scientists. There are subtler laws at work in the arena of the spirit world; the inner realm of consciousness marches to a different drummer.

Mind reading is a gift of the masters, but this need not concern the average person seeking their guidance in leading a more spiritual life. This invasion of privacy is not undertaken by masters unless it is necessary, and you have more cause for alarm in this area when dealing with a non-spiritual natural psychic who is able to tune in to your thoughts. Masters seldom abuse the powers they have and, in fact, do not even exhibit them until they have received a God-given sanction to do so. Should such an abuse occur through a lapse into the ego-ruled world of maya, all powers would be revoked. Patanjali warned against the seeking of powers lest they, and not communion with God, become the goal.

* *Shanti* means peace.

Modern Miracles—Metaphysical to Medical

Religious miracles are not confined to ages past and may be evidenced periodically in contemporary America, perhaps in substantiation of the biblical quote "Except ye see signs and wonders, ye will not believe" (John 4:48). In July, 1972, New Orleans, Louisiana, was host to a "weeping madonna"—a statue whose glass eyes so profusely welled with tears that fluid dripping from the tip of her nose could be clearly photographed.

One of two of its kind in the world, the Pilgrim Statue of Fatima was carved out of cedar under the guidance of Sister Lucy, the only survivor of the three children who claimed they witnessed the 1917 apparition of the Virgin Mary in Portugal.

Thousands of persons viewed the weeping statue during its ten-day stay in New Orleans, and the authenticity of the miracle was confirmed by the assistant chancellor of the archdiocese, the Reverend Lanaux Rareshide. He stated that the Church does not confirm such occurrences without thorough investigations to prevent the possibility of fraud or exploitation of believers.

No lesser miracle, at least from the viewpoint of a writer, was involved in the creation of *Jonathan Livingston Seagull*, a metaphysical story about a seagull. The ninety-three-page best-seller was written by Richard Bach, a former pilot whose previous writings were confined to the subject of aviation, and according to Bach, *Jonathan* was not written by him, but by "a Voice," aided by a vision.

Bach's introduction to *Jonathan* came on a foggy night in the early 1960s while walking along a canal in Belmont Shore, California, asking himself how he was going to pay the rent. Not expecting an answer, he was startled by the sound of a male voice, close by and not his own, that answered, "Jonathan Livingston Seagull." More than a little bewildered and a bit frightened, Bach rushed home, sat down at his desk, and invited the Voice to return.

Suddenly he saw a small solitary seagull flying over a very bright blue sea. Bach insists he knew the vision wasn't for his enjoyment alone, so he began writing what he saw and heard. After about ten pages the vision disappeared as abruptly as it had come, and Bach filed the unfinished manuscript away and forgot about it.

Eight years later he awoke at five o'clock one morning to find that the Voice and vision had returned. Again he wrote, and again the vision vanished. Bolder now, Bach invited the Voice back two more times before *Jonathan* was completed. He illustrated the tiny volume with seagull paintings done by a friend, submitted it to several publishers, and received rejection notices from all of them.

An editor at The Macmillan Company later sent a routine letter to Bach asking if he had any uncommitted manuscripts to show, and the result is now publishing history. Bach tightened the manuscript and replaced the seagull paintings with photographs. In keeping with the mysterious circumstances of this book, a friend he visited just happened to have a trunkful of seagull photos, which couldn't have been more appropriate had they been planned for use in the volume.

Without publicity backing from the publisher, the sale of *Jonathan Livingston Seagull* started slowly, then began picking up as one person told another . . . and another . . . and another. A year and a half later, word-of-mouth praise had mushroomed the book's sales to 200,000 copies. By July, 1972, nearly a half-million copies had been sold.

Although the success of *Jonathan* has made Richard Bach a rich man, he is reluctant to claim authorship and credits the work to God. He has publicly stated that "I feel that if I suddenly started taking credit for *Jonathan,* I'd be struck down by some lightning bolt as soon as I stepped outside." He adds, "I think all I was concerned about was that *Jonathan* was written and available to people who are right for it." As for all that money, Bach claims the Voice said, "Fine, go ahead and take the money, Bach, and buy an airplane."

Having great reverence for the Voice, he bought a 1947 Republic Seabee, a long-winged amphibian, from a man who knew nothing about Bach or his book. Airplane-owners are a sentimental breed, and as the former owner was viewing the plane for the last time, he said: "It's such a pretty thing. It looks kind of like a big seagull, doesn't it?"

Chief debunkers of supposed miracles have long been the scientists who believe only that which can be duplicated and proved in the laboratory. Now, in something akin to a miracle, they are shelving their skepticism and studying the yogis of India in an attempt to learn more about the real nature of man. To their credit, these scientists admit that advanced yogis demonstrate the ability to control bodily processes that the medical profession has always believed were involuntary and beyond our conscious control.

Biofeedback Training

Biofeedback training intrigued only a handful of scientists just four or five years ago; now it is being called one of the most important discoveries of our time. Should biofeedback training realize its purported potential, it could well create broad and sweeping changes that outdistance anyone's wildest dreams in medicine, education, industry, rehabilitation, and many other fields.

Biofeedback utilizes electronics in its mind-over-matter, or mind-over-body, training techniques. The key to the system is the recent discovery that the involuntary nervous system can be voluntarily controlled. Once a subject's internal processes, such as heart rate or blood pressure, are translated by powerful amplifiers into the blinking of lights, sound blips, or the fluctuations of a needle on a dial, the average ordinary person is able to influence these internal processes simply by thinking about it and willing it to be so. In other words, once a man is able to see his brain activity on a chart or graph, once he is able to watch his heart via these monitoring devices, he can learn to control them.

The medical implications of this concept are staggering. Clinical treatment of patients with biofeedback methods has been conducted at Maimonides Medical Center in Brooklyn, New York, in which diaphragmatic breathing has been taught to asthmatic children and adults with pulmonary insufficiency. Epileptics and cerebral palsy patients have been taught to control muscle spasms without drugs, and stroke and multiple sclerosis patients have been at least partially rehabilitated.

Psychologists at the University of Colorado Medical Center in Denver have reported that feedback therapy cured some patients who had suffered from muscle tension headaches for an average of nine years. And at Emory University in Atlanta, Georgia, biofeedback training has been channeled to aid the physically handicapped. Patients were taught to activate individual motor nerve cells out of the tens of thousands in a spinal cord, producing rhythmic "drumbeats" in a loudspeaker connected to a nerve fiber. This has led to the development of more efficient prosthetic devices for the handicapped and to an artificial breathing machine controlled by nerve impulses in a patient's chest.

Feedback proponents envision a future when cancer patients, as well as those with other tumors or warts, would starve these growths through blood-flow control, when essential hypertension patients would be taught to lower their own blood pressure, and when ulcer patients would consciously control the flow of gastric juices. Incidentally, one negative application of biofeedback training has already cropped up to assist draft dodgers, who are taught to mentally elevate their blood pressure to pathological levels.

Modern technology is very nearly outpacing our ability to comprehend it, assimilate it, and discard those former truths that no longer apply. The lag time between total disbelief, new evidence, and a reevaluation of old concepts is often so short that it embarrasses the experts. In early 1972 the prestigious and conventional American Medical Association was labeling acupuncture, the ancient Chinese medical art that uses thin needles inserted in specified parts of the body to alleviate pain and illness, as "arcane quackery." By mid-1972, however, the A.M.A. was most interested in studying this Oriental technique.

Heart specialist Paul Dudley White traveled to China to witness acupuncture anesthesia, and four U.S. Public Health Service doctors, acting on their own, have asked the Chinese for permission to enter China to study acupuncture. By the time this book is in print, acupuncture may well be an accepted procedure carrying the blessing of the A.M.A.

Wonders in Genetics

We are on the threshold of medical and scientific advances so reminiscent of the nightmare envisioned by Aldous Huxley and science fiction that they challenge credibility. The science of genetic engineering may be able in the foreseeable future to produce life through cloning, a process that will result in the production of genetic carbon copies of existing human beings. Babies have been fertilized in test tubes, though no embryo has yet lived beyond twenty-nine days.

Should cloning become a reality, a single body cell, which has a nucleus containing forty-six characteristic-determining chromosomes, could be chemically stimulated to produce an exact duplicate of the person from whom the cell was taken. This cell reportedly would be implanted into an artificial womb or in the uterus of a woman who would not be its mother, only a temporary host. The new life would have only one parent, the man or woman from whom the original cell was taken. Technically, we could then produce five hundred or a thousand or a million Einsteins, Beethovens —or Hitlers. Although cloning is not yet a reality, it is a distinct possibility for the near future, a possibility that many experts in science, religion, and philosophy view as an indication that our technology has outdistanced our wisdom.

Medical science has and is producing what would seem to be physiological miracles, particularly when viewed in the context of what medicine consisted of even thirty years ago, before the pill, Salk vaccine, and various transplant techniques were developed. Science is also broadening its horizons in matters of the mind—how the mind works, what influences the way we think, and the ultimate potential of this fantastic computerlike instrument.

Telepathic Invasion of Minds during Sleep

Science is now substantiating such an unlikely circumstance as the fact that even your dreams are influenced by the minds of other people. The

Maimonides Medical Center in Brooklyn has conducted experiments through its Dream Laboratory involving twelve thousand people to shed more scientific light on the dream state. According to the Miamonides Dream Laboratory Research Director, Dr. Stanley Krippner, "We consequently know that not everything you dream comes from your own inner consciousness. Some part of it can be projected to you from other people."

In these experiments a subject went to sleep for six consecutive nights at the center where technicians monitored him with special equipment that told them when he was sleeping. Forty-five miles away, in Port Chester, New York, the Grateful Dead, a well-known rock group, was putting on a series of performances for audiences of about two thousand every night.

Without warning or prior publicity the audience each night was asked to take part in the experiment. Their help was solicited by flashing a series of messages on the screen behind the performers. The message said: "You are about to participate in an ESP experiment. In a few seconds you will see a picture. Try using your ESP to 'send' this picture to Malcolm Bessent. He will try to dream about this picture. Malcolm Bessent is now at the Maimonides Dream Laboratory in Brooklyn." Then a different art print was projected onto the screen each night for fifteen minutes.

Back at the Dream Laboratory, Bessent was awakened after each dream and asked to tell what the dream was about. His answers were recorded and numbered in sequence. The prints and transcripts of the dreams were then given to two independent judges who did not know the order in which the prints had been shown, and these judges were asked to determine whether they could match the dreams to the prints.

In four out of six cases the judges were able to match the dreams with the prints, the dream occasionally mirroring the print very closely. When Scralian's painting *The Seven Spinal Chakras* was projected, the subject dreamed about "an energy box" and "a spinal column," both recognizable components of the painting.

Unknown to the audience, another sleeping subject who slept at home was also a part of the experiment. His dreams correlated to the prints only one time out of the six. According to Dr. Krippner, "It's obvious from this experiment and others we've conducted over the last seven years that people can actually invade each other's minds telepathically during sleep. But exactly how the invasions take place we don't yet know."

Since the unannounced sleeper scored less impressively than the one the audience knew about, it would seem that intentionality on the part of the agent is important, Dr. Krippner pointed out.

Since 1965 Dr. Krippner's Dream Laboratory has published more than one hundred articles on extrasensory perception in dreams in medical, psychological, psychiatric, and parapsychological journals. Dr. Krippner has also traveled to Russia to observe Soviet research at the Institute of Technical Parapsychology. He notes that the main difference between the American and the Russian approaches is that the thrust of American research is on simply proving the existence of ESP and PK (psychokinesis), whereas the Soviets fully accept the actuality of these phenomena. Russian research seeks practical applications of these phenomena and an understanding of how they work.

Parapsychology is concerned with phenomena usually considered outside the realm of orthodox psychology and deals primarily with extrasensory perception and psychokinesis. ESP refers to information received other than through the usual senses and includes clairvoyance, visions or second sight, and telepathy (mind-to-mind communication). PK is the term applied when objects seemingly move by themselves or are made to move by the will of a "sensitive."

Psychic phenomena are fully accepted in Russia, and the Soviet Union has some six major parapsychological research centers and a dozen minor ones. The United States has approximately an equal number, the main difference between them being that those in Russia are all government funded and supported. In the United States only one of these centers receives any federal financial support. In addition, the majority of Russian scientists support parapsychological research and can accept the new concepts that arise from it.

The handful of American scientists and medical doctors who admit belief in psychic phenomena do so at the risk of their professional reputation. Dr. Shafica Karagulla, neuropsychiatrist and author of *Breakthrough to Creativity: Your Higher Sense Perception*, relates in her book cases of numerous medical doctors who utilize what she terms higher sense perception in their practices. Her term, which she abbreviates HSP, would seem to correlate with the phrase "supersensory perception or extraordinary sense" perception preferred by anthropologist Margaret Mead, a longstanding member of the American Society for Psychical Research.

Some of these professionals studied by Dr. Karagulla have the ability to know intuitively or actually "see" through the gift of second sight, the illnesses of their patients. Others "know," regardless of where they are, which patients are ill and need their help. Many claim to have the ability to "see" the energy vortices along the spine which correlate with the chakras discussed in Chapter 4. Some of these doctors are world-famous diagnosticians because of their unique talents, yet none of them have the courage to risk the incredulity of their peers or their professional standing by admitting their unusual abilities. Such is the status of psychic phenomena in the United States.

On the other hand, the research findings of several other countries are seemingly beginning to substantiate the ancient yoga concept of man as an integral link with the entire cosmos, a part of all life on earth and in the universe. This view of man accepts his complete interaction, via the physical and astral bodies and the mind, with the planets, the environment, and all other forms of life: human, animal, and plant.

Science Substantiates Yoga

Yogis have, for thousands of years, maintained that man has a physical body composed of matter and an astral body composed of a subtler substance beyond man's range of vision. The astral body is said to be an exact duplicate of the physical except that it has fewer limitations than the physical body. Man's physical body is nourished and maintained through food, water, and oxygen, these elements being distributed throughout the entire system by means of the circulatory system. The physical body is laced with a network of arteries and veins to carry out the work of the circulatory system.

The astral body is sustained by means of prana obtained in the oxygen we breathe. This prana, or vital energy, is then distributed throughout the astral body by the nadis—some 72,000 of them—which were discussed in Chapter 4. The physical and astral bodies are connected by a cord that is severed upon death, at which time the astral body leaves the physical, but does not disintegrate, and continues to exist on another plane.

Also, according to the yogis, the physical body is the vehicle that uses the five known senses of sight, hearing, taste, touch, and smell. The sixth sense, or senses, which includes telepathy, clairvoyance, and all extrasensory perceptions, is the province of the astral body. All plants, animals, and men have both a physical and an astral body, and both bodies are controlled by the mind.

In the late 1930s a Russian electrician, Semyon Kirlian, and his wife, Valentina, invented a method of photography that photographed the energy field surrounding all forms of life. A leaf so photographed showed colored flarelike projections emanating from the leaf. Each species of life, they discovered, has its own specific pattern of projections. The Kirlians' continuing experiments revealed that their photographs indicated the state of health of life forms photographed, with disease showing in the photos before symptoms were noted.

For example, two leaves were photographed from the exact same species of plant. Both leaves were removed at the same time, one leaf from one plant and the other leaf from another plant of the same species. The photographs showed distinctly different flare patterns projecting from the leaves, and the photographs were repeated again and again with the same results. The Kirlians were then told that one leaf came from a plant infected with a disease that would eventually kill it. Though no symptoms had yet appeared on either plant or leaf, the energy field, or astral body, of the plant already revealed the effect of the disease.

Clairvoyants, mediums, some advanced yogis, and several of the doctors studied by Dr. Shafica Karagulla assert that they have the ability to see the aura enveloping all life forms. The aura has been described as a luminescence surrounding the physical body which, like the Kirlian photographs, showed impending illness or disease as a weaker luminescence in the area that would later be the site of the problem. In view of the Kirlian experiments, it may be that the aura does not actually exist, but what appears to be the aura is actually the flarelike projections from the astral, or energy, body.

Persons claiming to see auras report that even if a limb is amputated, they see that limb intact in the aura or energy field. The Kirlian photographs also record the whole energy body, even though a part is missing. Medical doctors have long been baffled by amputees who still experience pain in a missing limb and are inclined to relegate such complaints to hysteria or hypochondria. Perhaps future scientific research may prove that this pain does still exist in the astral body and translates itself to the physical in some as yet unknown manner.

Patents on the Kirlian instruments were turned over to their state government where the parapsychological climate thirty years ago was much like it is in the United States at this time. Little was done with Kirlian photography until the more favorable parapsychological atmosphere of the 1960s emerged and government funds were channeled into research on it. Now, coupled with the other developments that are emerging from that country, the Kirlians' discoveries may someday shed a great deal of light on many subjects not completely understood at this time.

Yogis and philosophers, and in later periods, positive thinkers and Christian Scientists, have linked the way we think to the way we actually are. Negative emotions such as anger, hatred, and basic negativity produce correspondingly dire circumstances in our physical bodies and external environment. The Kirlian photographs prove that these negative states of mind produce changes in the human energy field that can be photographed. When vital energy in the astral body is diminished for any length of time, it is soon mirrored in the physical body as illness.

On one occasion the Kirlians had scheduled a demonstration of their equipment for some of Russia's leading scientists and were most anxious about the results. Testing the equipment before their distinguished guests arrived, Kirlian was disconcerted to find that the photograph of his hand showed minimal, indistinct, and unusual projections, instead of the clear, colorful light emanations he expected.

When the guests arrived, photographs of the guests' hands showed the normal projections the Kirlians had come to anticipate. Time and time again, the machinery performed erratically when being tested before a major demonstration for high-ranking scientific dignitaries. Eventually, the Kirlians began to realize that the machine was working fine; it was merely reflecting their own tension, worry, and anxiety about the impending demonstration.

Kirlian photographs clearly indicate that the energy body is instantly affected by fatigue, illness, emotions, attitudes, and alcohol, and that in these conditions the energy pattern changes, and more vital energy is dissipated from the body.

Kirlian Photography and Astrology . . . Reincarnation

Through Kirlian photography there may be an impending breakthrough in, among other things, astrology. During periods of sunspot eruptions the Kirlian photographs reflected this activity. Since this form of photography is dealing with the energy, or astral, body, perhaps the pull of the planets is exerted on the astral body rather than on the physical. Soviet scientists have also photographed plants and animals in the process of death. Gradually, as the physical body died, these scientists observed and photographed sparks and flares of the energy body shooting off into space, swimming away, and disappearing. Biological field detectors placed at a distance from the now dead body continued to detect pulsating force fields. They speculate that this pulsation could be issuing from the detached astral body, an occurrence suggestive of continued life on another plane.

Acupuncture and the Astral Body

Acupuncture has been used by the Chinese for thousands of years to cure disease and to control pain. Although they are convinced of its effectiveness, and it is a standard medical procedure in that country, the Chinese cannot explain why acupuncture, a technique in which thin needles are inserted into the body at various points, is successful.

Though not as common as in China, acupuncture is also being used in Russia. What we have called the astral body or the energy body is termed bioplasma in Russia, and it is presumed to be a fourth state of matter that is in constant interaction with other states of matter. One of the greatest problems in acupuncture has always been to determine the exact location of the treatment points on the skin, which measure less than a millimeter in width.

Using the Kirlian equipment as a guide (the flares occur at the acupuncture points), the Russians have invented a device called the tobiscope, displayed at Expo 67 in Montreal, which detects the acupuncture points. The tobiscope is about the size of a small flashlight. When this device is slowly moved across a person's face, its light flashes off and on, the on position signaling an acupuncture point. Good health is indicated when this light is bright, and a dim light indicates that there is a current or future health problem.

The tobiscope is said to measure the body's "bioplasmic energy." When readings are obtained from several acupuncture points, the flow of bioplasmic energy throughout the body can be determined. This measurement of the bioplasmic system, which many Russian scientists feel will eventually be recognized to be of equal importance as the circulatory, lymphatic, and nervous systems, can be used to predict and treat disease. Russian physicians, however, substitute other means of stimulating the acupuncture points in preference to the Chinese needles. They work on the appropriate points with massage, ointments, lotions, weak pulses of electricity, injected chemicals, and even, in the case of epileptic seizures, laser beams.

The Russian approach to acupuncture may be a key to understanding why some spontaneous cures for various ills occur seemingly through yoga practice. Although I have stated throughout this book that yoga does not cure disease, yoga postures and exercises exert pressure on all parts of the human body. As the student progresses in yoga practice, the postures are held for increasingly longer periods of time. Since the body supposedly contains some nine hundred acupuncture points, obviously some of these points will be involved, or receive more than average pressure and stimulation during the holding of various postures.

The ancient Chinese physicians conceptualized a life energy running through the body, an energy that resembles the Russian concept of bioplasma and the yoga concept of prana. The Chinese further believed that this life energy was thrown out of balance by such internal conditions as disease and emotions as well as such diverse external conditions as the seasons, the changing phases of the moon and tides, thunderstorms, strong winds, and even noise levels (stress?). Should this imbalance not be corrected, the Chinese maintained that illness was inevitable.

If the Chinese concept is an accurate one—a concept that is being pursued diligently in Russia and increasingly in the United States—we may soon find that the pressure applied through yoga postures does, indeed, have a curative effect.

Perhaps acupuncture research may also someday prove scientifically why yoga practice increases psychic ability. Yoga masters, through control of the prana in their systems, have been known for thousands of years to possess extraordinary powers of extrasensory perception, telepathy, and other abilities, as mentioned earlier in this chapter. This ability is generally attributed to stimulation of the pituitary and pineal glands. These powers remain only so long as the yogi uses them for the good of mankind; they are revoked if they are abused.

It may be that the yogi augments the vital life energy, or prana, in the system through his controlled breathing, and assures its balanced distribution throughout his body (or bodies—physical and astral) through the various physical postures. Thus, since the astral or energy body has been shown by Kirlian photography to be affected by emotional states and attitudes, any ego-directed or impure attitudes could create an imbalance in the energy body and thus lessen or destroy these powers and abilities. East and West seem to be closer than they have ever been, and we may soon see the mysteries of yogic powers explained and verified in the laboratory.

Meditation

Another aspect of yoga currently being probed under the microscope of science is meditation, the last step on the yogi's road to samadhi. Meditation has always been an integral part of yoga, but we live in a technological era in which people are geared to being told "how to do it." Since meditation is an abstract concept, and also because it involves seemingly unproductive time, many yoga teachers and students disregard it.

This aspect of yoga, however, has been organized and westernized into a system called transcendental meditation (TM), a system stripped of the discipline of exercise and one that requires no specific life-style or spiritual allegiance. TM made its American debut several years ago when Mia Farrow and the Beatles trekked to India to learn the technique from its innovator, Maharishi Mahesh Yogi. Although the giggling guru's penchant for publicity and commercialization turned many people off, the concept behind his system has had growing acceptance with both the lay public and the scientific community.

Since its inception in 1965, the International Meditation Society, the Los Angeles–based nonprofit organization that teaches TM, has reportedly trained more than 150,000 Americans in the technique, with an additional 5,000 people being added each month. Among the converts are otherwise conservative businessmen, housewives, students, scientists, and teachers.

Transcendental meditation has been defined as "a method of allowing the mind to be drawn automatically to the deepest and most refined level of thinking." Meditation in many minds is confused with prayer, but there are quite specific differences. In prayer the one praying is asking for something; in meditation the meditator waits for an answer.

Instruction in organized transcendental meditation is available in most large cities in the United States. During these training periods, which include four two-hour periods, each person is assigned a personal mantra which the International Meditation Society calls "the vehicle that allows meditation to take place."

As discussed in Chapter 4, the mantra is a combination of Sanskrit phrases, and I.M.S., as well as all yogis, stresses that the mantra must be kept secret. Skeptics of the organization contend that this secrecy is an effort to assure that no one has a magical mantra without first paying the course fee of $75 for adults and $45 for students.

Meditators sit upright in a chair with eyes closed and listen to the instructor chant the mantra. The meditator then takes up the mantra himself, first aloud and then silently. The muscles of the body relax during meditation and may even twitch involuntarily, the head sometimes slumping forward, the whole picture suggestive of sleep. Meditators claim, however, that their minds remain acutely aware of all outside stimuli, such as noises and movements in the room, and that the process requires no effort.

Each person's meditation experience is unique, but one practiced meditator describes her experience like this: "You close your eyes, and after a few minutes the mantra just floats into your consciousness. Sometimes noises or mundane daydreams may distract you, but then you find your mind wandering back to the mantra. You feel a deep sense of rest and alertness pass through your mind and body." TM devotees say the meditative response begins as soon as the mind turns to the mantra, though no one seems to know or care what triggers this response.

Meditators are urged to meditate twenty minutes each morning and evening, and they credit the system with producing freedom from tension, mental well-being, heightened energy and creativity, and the ability to function more effectively in the high-pressure rat race of everyday life. They report a feeling of harmony with their surroundings, a less critical attitude toward other people, and less anxiety.

Science Looks at TM

Initially skeptical about the claims of TM, scientists at hospitals and universities around the country are now investigating its potential as therapy for drug addicts, prisoners, and mental patients as well as treatment for certain diseases. Cardiologist Dr. Herbert Benson, assistant professor of medicine at Harvard Medical School, and physiologist R. K. Wallace have conducted experiments with thirty-six meditators. The volunteer meditators had been utilizing the technique for varying lengths of time—one month being the shortest and nine years the longest.

The results of this experiment, which were reported in the *Wall Street Journal*, demonstrated the following results:

> During meditation, the subjects' blood pressures were found to be low, their heart and respiration rates slowed, oxygen consumption was reduced, and their blood lactate levels (which some scientists believe is related to anxiety) decreased markedly. The meditators also showed heightened alpha brain wave activity—normally seen in a rested, relaxed state. The physiological responses during meditation differed from those generally observed during waking, sleeping and hypnotic states, the researchers reported.
>
> Dr. Benson explains that stress produces in most people what scientists term the "fight or flight" response: Blood pressure and heart rate zoom, respiration speeds up, and the blood flow to the muscles is markedly increased. Constantly turning on this response may lead to permanent high blood pressure, Dr. Benson theorizes.
>
> "The meditational response appears to be exactly the opposite of the fight or flight response," he says. Noting that one-third of all adults in this country suffer from definite or borderline hypertension (high blood pressure), he is investigating whether by lowering blood pressure during the day by meditating, "we may be able to prevent and even treat high blood pressure." He is currently training hypertensive patients to meditate, to see if TM can successfully lower their blood pressure.
>
> Dr. Benson and other scientists have also been successful in altering such "involuntary" physiological functions as heart rate and blood pressure using "Biofeedback," or mental conditioning, techniques. Dr. Benson, however, believes the physiological changes observed during meditation are unique to meditation and haven't been produced through biofeedback methods.

Meditation and Drug Abuse

In a separate study the Benson-Wallace team is investigating TM's effectiveness in combating drug abuse. A questionnaire relating to drug habits was distributed to 1,862 meditators. The results showed that as the practice of meditation continued, the subjects progressively decreased their use of drugs. After twenty-one months, for example, the number of subjects using marijuana dropped from 80 percent to 12 percent, and the number of LSD users went from 48 percent to 3 percent. Though most of the subjects felt that meditation was instrumental in their decreasing or halting drug use, Dr. Benson termed the study "inconclusive, since the experiment wasn't controlled."

He found the implications so promising, however, that he is now conducting a two-year study of the drug-use patterns of ten thousand high-school juniors, some of whom will be taught to meditate. Dr. Benson believes that since no one has yet solved the drug problem, "meditation deserves further investigation to see whether it is a nonchemical alternative to drug use."

Other researchers are studying the effects of meditation on psychiatric patients, prisoners, and U.S. Army personnel. And meditation may soon be a subject taught in the nation's schools. The National Institutes of Mental Health, of the U.S. Department of Health, Education, and Welfare, recently awarded the I.M.S. $21,540 to train one hundred secondary-school teachers to teach meditation in high schools. In one school where meditation has been taught, in Eastchester, New York, the superintendent of schools reports that "meditators get better grades, stop using drugs, are more outgoing, and get along better with their parents, teachers, and friends."

How to Meditate

Though all the research findings aren't in yet, evidence seems to be mounting that meditation, whether organized or not, does provide profound benefits. In the physical, mental, and spiritual developmental system of yoga, meditation provides the spiritual element; without meditation, yoga is simply not yoga. While transcendental meditation has been systematized and made easy for the Western world, it is not necessary to go through their training program in order to meditate.

Following yoga postures and breathing exercises, Steps 3 and 4 in Patanjali's astanga-yoga (see Chapter 4), comes sense withdrawal (Step 5), concentration (Step 6), and finally meditation (Step 7), which leads to samadhi, the eighth and final step. After performing the postures, allow ten minutes for relaxation, during which you mentally tell each part of your body to relax. Following this relaxation period, while you are alone or at a time when you will not be interrupted, sit on the floor or a mat in any comfortable cross-legged position or in the full or half lotus when these become comfortable.

Now, starting with the feet, mentally withdraw all feeling and sensation from the feet. This is Step 5, sense withdrawal. Mentally disassociate yourself from your feet. Continue, withdrawing feeling and sensation from the legs, the lower trunk, the upper trunk, the hands and arms, and finally the scalp, the skin of the forehead, cheeks, eyelids, mouth, and tongue.

At this point your consciousness should be centered completely on your mind. You may even have the feeling that the mind is larger and more expanded. Now use your mind to concentrate—Step 6—on the universal mantra Om. Close your eyes and say aloud, "Om." When the sound of the mantra has become so familiar that you can hear it in your mind without actually saying it, discontinue saying it aloud, and instead repeat it to yourself mentally.

Don't expect anything to happen at first, and don't allow yourself to become tense while waiting. Eventually it will come.

10

MATURITY

Someone once said that humans are children for so long that they never get over it. Yoga views man in a more hopeful light, a light nevertheless in which hope is tempered with a good bit of realism. As mentioned in the first chapter, instead of assuming that humanity reaches maturity, along with legal age, at twenty-one, we feel that it usually takes longer than that. Unfortunately, by the time most people reach the mid-forties, and hopefully achieve some wisdom and maturity, their bodies have been abused and misused to the extent that they are a problem.

No one can really appreciate life, maturity, or anything else if the physical body is a discomfort and distraction. The yoga postures, the breathing methods, and the insights into the human condition outlined in previous chapters, if applied, should prevent premature bodily deterioration and help restore health if damage has already been done. The physical body *can* be changed.

Maturity is something else. The dictionary defines a mature person as one who is fully developed in body and mind, a definition I reject because it assumes that knowledge is a static thing, instead of progressive, growing, ever-changing; it ignores the fact that the truths of yesterday may well be unseated tomorrow. Preferable, I think, is Louis Binstock's definition, in *The Power of Maturity*, that says, "Maturity is not a state of being; it is a state of becoming. You may say to yourself: 'I am not a human being; I am a human becoming.' "

The Power of Maturity

The mature person has the mental flexibility to discard the beliefs and emotional postures that no longer have validity. Maturity, like relaxation, is highly recommended, but how-to literature on both subjects is often phrased in such technical terms that it is of little real value to the average person.

Further complicating the quest for maturity is the erroneous assumption that psychological age, which represents one's degree of maturity or immaturity, is somehow linked to chronological age. In *The Mature Mind* H. A. Overstreet stated that "not all adults are adult. Many who look grown-up on the outside may be childish on the inside. Others who look childish on the outside may be surprisingly mature on the inside. Whether a person is average, advanced, or retarded in his mental, emotional, and social growth may be the concealed reason—and the chief reason—why his adult relationships with his world are as they are."

The Mature Mind was written in 1949, and Overstreet noted in it that "the concept of psychological age has only begun to enter our common consciousness." The book sold more than half a million copies, an indication of the growing awareness of the public that there was room for improvement in the human condition. The popularity of psychoanalysis further underscored the fact that we are a nation of people with problems that we are unable to solve by ourselves.

Psychoanalysis has undoubtedly helped many people, unfortunately at a very high cost in terms of time and financial outlay for the patients. Problems are not restricted to the wealthy, but generally speaking, only the wealthy can afford psychiatry. Until the last few years there was little help available to the average person who didn't quite understand himself, or for the person who was mentally healthy and stable but who felt the need to nurture his growing maturity to an even greater understanding of himself and other people.

Transactional Analysis

Transactional analysis seems to have filled a vast void in providing the tools for better self-knowledge. *I'm OK, You're OK*, written by Dr. Thomas A. Harris, explains the subject in terms anyone can understand.

Transactional analysis (TA) is a system of sorting out and understanding human behavior that does not require the long period of "time on the couch" and correspondingly high cost of traditional psychoanalysis. Its proponents also feel it is more effective because TA uses simplified language stripped of the mumbo-jumbo of psychiatry. Because of its simplicity, TA is used successfully even with the severely mentally retarded.

Transactional analysis is a new breakthrough, one that confronts the individual with the fact that he is responsible for what happens in the future, no matter what happened in the past. In a nutshell TA is the concept that each personality has three components—Parent, Adult, and Child, these words being capitalized to emphasize the fact that they have different meanings in TA from their meanings when used in everyday conversation. All three are necessary for an integrated, stable personality, and all three contain different sets of data that affect human behavior.

The Child is the part of us that contains all feelings and emotions. When you feel hurt, it is the Child within that hurts. Data in the Child has been recorded since birth, and even people born into loving and encouraging families have what Dr. Harris calls a Not OK Child position, a position that causes many behavior problems. The Not OK Child position is the inevitable result of having been small, dependent, and inadequate to control one's circumstances, the feeling of being two feet tall in a world of six-footers. The feelings experienced then are recorded in the tape recorder of the brain and replayed throughout life whenever people feel inadequate to the situation or "backed into a corner." Your Not OK Child feels now as you felt then.

The OK Child is that part of you that has fun, creates, and has the urge to learn and explore new things and ideas. The OK Child is in charge whenever you enjoy a good belly laugh.

Your Parent data consists of those things you learned from your actual parents (or parent substitute), the do's and don'ts—things such as "You must always brush your teeth after meals," "Never get in debt," and "You will always find that the best people are Methodists" (or Catholics or Jews, whatever your actual parents thought). Tip-offs to Parent data are words such as "always," "must," "never," and "should" in a statement, particularly when emphasized with the extended index finger. Not all data recorded in the Parent is accurate or up-to-date.

Parent data were recorded as the gospel truth at a time when the youngster looked to the actual parents as total security and total knowledge, when the child had no corrective information. If the actual parents were extremely prejudiced, bigoted, or narrow-minded, the Parent facet of the developing personality will also carry this data. Because the Parent data were recorded as truth, it is the function of the Adult within us all to examine that data, as well as all other facets of life, to determine what squares with reality.

Through the Adult, which begins to develop at about ten months of age, people learn the difference between life as it was taught and demonstrated to him (Parent), life as he felt it or wished it or fantasied it

(Child), and life as he figures it out for himself (Adult). The goal of transactional analysis is to free up each person's Adult from the trouble-making influences and demands of his Parent and Child, to get the individual off the hook of the past.

Yoga and Maturity

A discussion of maturity in a book that is basically about yoga may seem strange, particularly since the subject is rarely mentioned in a yoga class. I think they should be viewed together for several reasons.

In the first place yoga is a system of physical, mental, and spiritual development. Yoga develops unusual uses of the mind—for visualization, affirmation, concentration, and meditation—but mental development also means to use the mind in a mature manner. The immature mind sees the world and everything in it only in relationship to itself, whereas the maturity concept, and the basis of yoga, strives to see the whole picture, the whole universe, in perspective as unified, related, and integrated.

One of the goals of yoga is a letting go of the ego principle, and one of the goals of maturity is increased awareness of the feelings, wishes, and rights of others. These two goals are stated in different terms, but they mean essentially the same thing.

Another reason to stress maturity is that we live in a world of such rapid change that only the mature person can hope to cope with the new facts, values, and ways of living that are emerging. The immature person, fixated in some past stage of development, can only become bewildered and lost in the culture that is reshaping itself in the last decades of the twentieth century.

One of the greatest problems facing the world at this time is the survival of our planet. Our individual transgressions, and those of our technological society, have abused our environments—both the personal environment of the human body and the larger planetary environment—to the point of almost no return. World governments are enforcing and will no doubt continue to enforce regulations geared to righting our planetary picture, but in the long run it will probably be the responsibility of each of our citizens, working in our immediate environment—our own bodies, families, and homes—that will ultimately decide the fate of our world. And only the mature will be able to see the larger picture.

Getting into yoga changes people. As they become more aware of the unity of the physical, mental, and spiritual components within themselves, they also become more aware of the unity in the outer, larger world. Instead of seeing themselves as separate and apart from the rest of humanity, they become more closely related, and there is an increased feeling of kinship with all forms of life. As we learn to appreciate ourselves more, there is a corresponding appreciation, empathy, and feeling of responsibility for other people.

Yoga means union . . . to yoke or to join. It is a way of getting yourself together, and it is also a way of bridging the gap between you and other people. Not everyone in yoga is completely mature, but as maturity is a process of becoming, yoga is also a process of becoming. Yoga is not a cure-all for the multiple ills of individuals or of the world, but it is certainly a step in the right direction.

Index